The *illustrated* lecture series

Hematology
and Immunology

D1227671

The *illustrated* lecture series

Neurology and Psychiatry	P. N. Plowman
Endocrinology and Metabolic Diseases	P. N. Plowman
Nephrology, Electrolyte Pathophysiology and Poisoning	P. N. Plowman
Haematology and Immunology	P. N. Plowman
Cardiology	T. J. Phillips, P. N. Plowman
Respiratory Medicine	P. N. Plowman
Alimentary Medicine and Tropical Diseases	P. N. Plowman, T. J. Phillips, S. J. Rose

In Preparation

Surgery

Anatomy

Obstetrics and Gynaecology

Pathology

Physiology

Ophthalmology

The *illustrated* lecture series

Hematology and Immunology

P. N. Plowman MA MD (Cantab) MRCP FRCR
Consultant Physician
St Bartholomew's Hospital and Medical College
London EC1 UK

MEDICAL EXAMINATION PUBLISHING COMPANY

Distributors in the United States & Canada:
Medical Examination Publishing Company
A Division of Elsevier Science Publishing Co., Inc.
52 Vanderbilt Avenue, New York, New York 10017

Copyright©1987 by John Wiley & Sons Ltd.
Baffins Lane, Chichester, Sussex, UK

ISBN 0 444 01266 4

Printed in Great Britain

Contents

Contents

Immunology

Preface

Haematology is one of the fundamental specialties in medicine and yet the mixed laboratory and clinical elements of the subject have made it difficult for the student to comprehend well. In this book, the text is linked to diagrams illustrating each important point and this particularly assists the student to understand and to memorise.

Immunology is no less important a subject with contributions to our understanding of diseases afflicting many viscera. It is not possible to produce an all-embracing manual on this topic here but the essentials of immunology to the clinician are explained and well illustrated.

P. N. Plowman

Publisher's Note

Modern medicine is now more interesting and challenging than ever before. Unfortunately, the subject is now so large that it presents a formidable task for students to encompass and for the practising physician to maintain an up-to-date knowledge.

This series of illustrated books represents an entirely new concept which we believe will open up a new method of medical teaching, adding an extra dimension which will keep the reader's interest alive and active throughout the whole syllabus of general medicine.

The most important feature of the book is the linkage and locking of prose with figures in such a way that illustrations (with repeated key phrases) reinforce the comprehension of the text at all stages as one proceeds through the pages. The content of the series also differs from many standard works in that not only does it bring in new sections on subjects such as coma, brain death, blood transfusion reactions, etc. omitted in older texts, but it also recognises that certain diseases (e.g. tertiary syphilis) no longer merit extensive description whilst other subjects (e.g. current successes in oncology) merit a more generous coverage.

This series, when completed and collected together, should comprise a uniquely illustrated textbook for the entire medical curriculum. Although primarily intended for the undergraduate student, these books should also prove substantially helpful to nurses, paramedics and social workers who are academically inclined, and offer a refresher course to the busy practitioner.

We have tried to make academic life for the student easier. We shall welcome criticisms, comments and suggestions from academics, students and other readers since we feel sure that these will help us to improve future editions.

Hematology

THE PERIPHERAL BLOOD INDICES

The circulating peripheral blood contains three types of corpuscle: The erythrocytes (the 'red cells'), the leucocytes (the 'white cells') and the thrombocytes (the platelets). All three types ultimately derive from red bone marrow precursor 'stem cells', and the circulating numbers of the mature corpuscles are usually tightly controlled by poorly understood homeostatic controls acting on these marrow stem cells.

The erythrocytes function to carry oxygen from the lungs to the peripheral tissues and owe this property to their intracellular haemoglobin content. Haemoglobin is a complicated molecule comprising a globin (protein) moiety consisting of four peptide chains, and a haem (iron-proto-porphyrin) moiety. The marrow stem cell (the erythroblast) contains no haemoglobin and haemoglobinisation takes place as the daughter cells pass through the normoblast stage.

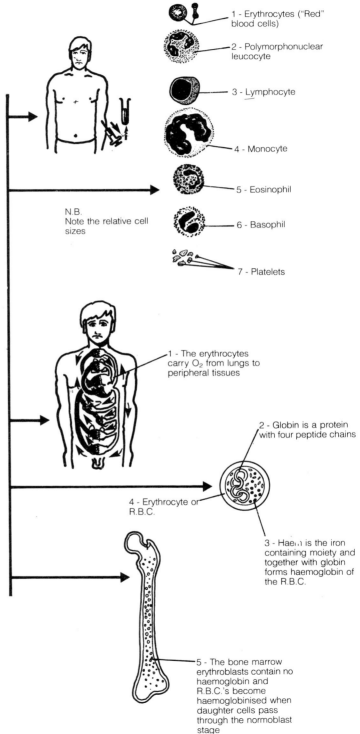

1 - Erythrocytes ("Red" blood cells)

2 - Polymorphonuclear leucocyte

3 - Lymphocyte

4 - Monocyte

5 - Eosinophil

6 - Basophil

7 - Platelets

N.B.
Note the relative cell sizes

1 - The erythrocytes carry O_2 from lungs to peripheral tissues

2 - Globin is a protein with four peptide chains

4 - Erythrocyte or R.B.C.

3 - Haem is the iron containing moiety and together with globin forms haemoglobin of the R.B.C.

5 - The bone marrow erythroblasts contain no haemoglobin and R.B.C.'s become haemoglobinised when daughter cells pass through the normoblast stage

3

After this stage of development the nucleus of the cell pyknoses and disappears leaving a reticulocyte (or immature erythrocyte) – recognisable due to the persistence of stainable ribonucleoprotein in the cytoplasm. Reticulocytes are normally found as 0.2–2.0% of the peripheral blood red cell count (24–84×10^9/l). The vast majority of peripheral blood red cells are mature erythrocytes.

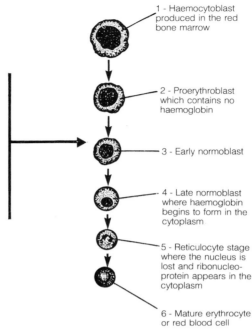

1 - Haemocytoblast produced in the red bone marrow

2 - Proerythroblast which contains no haemoglobin

3 - Early normoblast

4 - Late normoblast where haemoglobin begins to form in the cytoplasm

5 - Reticulocyte stage where the nucleus is lost and ribonucleoprotein appears in the cytoplasm

6 - Mature erythrocyte or red blood cell

An important functional investigation is the haemoglobin (Hb) concentration, (determined by the cyanomethaemoglobin optical density method). A normal adult man has an Hb of 13.5–18.0g/dl and a menstruating woman 11.5–16.5g/dl. Patients with lower Hb values are said to be anaemic. The **packed cell volume (PCV)** or haematocrit is another basic parameter expressed as the percentage (volume) occupied by the cell pellet in a blood specimen, (normal range men: 40–50%, women: 35–47%). The **mean cell haemoglobin concentration (MCHC)**, derived by division (Hb÷PCV) × 100, provides one indicator of red cell content of haemoglobin.

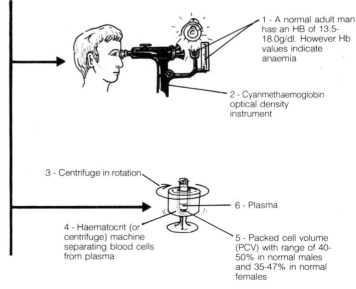

1 - A normal adult man has an HB of 13.5-18.0g/dl. However Hb values indicate anaemia

2 - Cyanmethaemoglobin optical density instrument

3 - Centrifuge in rotation

4 - Haematocrit (or centrifuge) machine separating blood cells from plasma

5 - Packed cell volume (PCV) with range of 40-50% in normal males and 35-47% in normal females

6 - Plasma

In the most commonly used automated blood cell counter, a blood cell suspension is passed through a small orifice across which a small electric current is flowing. By displacing some of the conducting fluid the cells raise the electrical resistance across the orifice. The passage of each cell thus produces a voltage pulse of short duration which is counted – its amplitude being proportional to the **mean cell volume (MCV** – normal range 76–96 fl).

Another red cell index that is readily available from such automated machinery is the **mean cell haemoglobin (MCH** – normal range 27–32 pg) and indeed this modern technology is highly sensitive to changes in red cell volume or haemoglobinisation.

Also, the machine red cell counting is far more precise than manual methods (normal range, men: 4.5–6.5 × 10^{12}/l, women: 3.9–5.6 × 10^{12}/l). This precision also extends to platelet counting which it is now possible to accurately and quickly quantify, (normal range: 150-450 x 10^9/l).

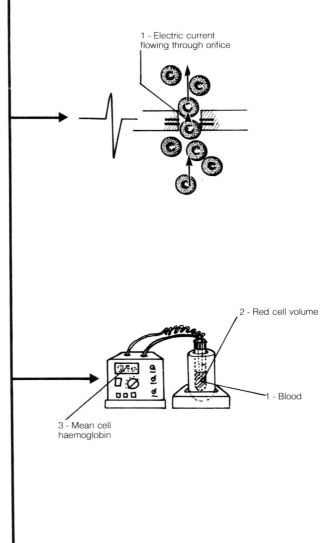

1 - Electric current flowing through orifice

2 - Red cell volume

1 - Blood

3 - Mean cell haemoglobin

The normal white cell count (4–11×10^9/l) is also obtainable from an electronic cell counter but the differential white cell count still relies on the examination of a blood film. The predominant leucocyte is the **neutrophil** (or polymorphonuclear granulocyte – normal range 2.0–7.5×10^9/l), which, with two other cell types containing cytopasmic granules (the **eosinophil** 00.4×10^9/l and the **basophil** 00.2×10^9/l) represent the end products of the 'myeloid series'. The parent of this cell line is the bone marrow **myeloblast** whose divisions and maturation stages in the marrow produce myelocytes and meta-myelocytes before the mature granulocytes are released into the blood. The neutrophil is the leucocyte most commonly associated with an acute inflammatory response and its numbers rise in acute infection, (neutrophil leucocytosis).

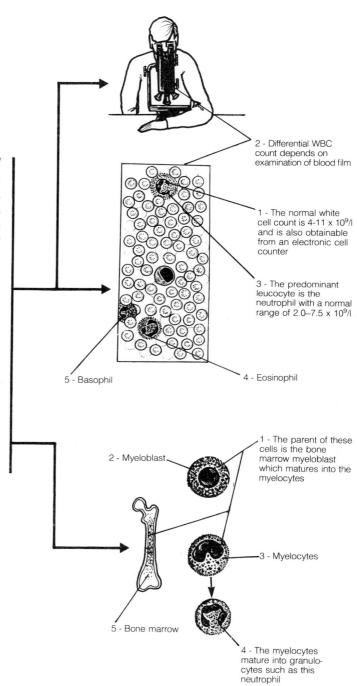

2 - Differential WBC count depends on examination of blood film

1 - The normal white cell count is 4-11 x 10^9/l and is also obtainable from an electronic cell counter

3 - The predominant leucocyte is the neutrophil with a normal range of 2.0–7.5 x 10^9/l

5 - Basophil

4 - Eosinophil

2 - Myeloblast

1 - The parent of these cells is the bone marrow myeloblast which matures into the myelocytes

3 - Myelocytes

5 - Bone marrow

4 - The myelocytes mature into granulocytes such as this neutrophil

The normal **lymphocyte** count is 1.0–3.5 × 10^9/l and the normal monocyte count 0–0.8 × 10^9/l. Lymphocytes mediate immune reactions (see immunology chapter), and the blood monocyte is the precursor of the peripheral tissue macrophage.

Examination of a well-spread, well-stained blood film remains the most important screening test for blood disease. Inspection of the blood film provides a check on the automated blood count. In addition, many blood disorders and minor vagaries in cell morphology which may not be associated with a significant alteration in **Hb, PCV** or total **leucocyte** or **platelet** counts may be diagnosed, (eg early megaloblastic anaemia, compensated haemolysis, lead poisoning, early lymphocytic or lymphoblastic leukaemia, infectious mononucleosis, agranulocytosis, eosinophilia, malarial or filarial parasitic inclusions, hereditary anomalies etc.).

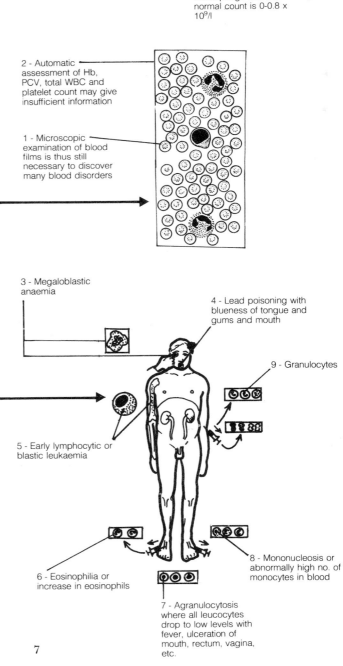

1 - Normal lymphocyte count is 1.0-3.5 x 10^9/l. Lymphocytes mediate immune reactions

2 - A blood monocyte here is the precursor of peripheral tissue macrophage and the normal count is 0-0.8 x 10^9/l

2 - Automatic assessment of Hb, PCV, total WBC and platelet count may give insufficient information

1 - Microscopic examination of blood films is thus still necessary to discover many blood disorders

3 - Megaloblastic anaemia

4 - Lead poisoning with blueness of tongue and gums and mouth

9 - Granulocytes

5 - Early lymphocytic or blastic leukaemia

8 - Mononucleosis or abnormally high no. of monocytes in blood

6 - Eosinophilia or increase in eosinophils

7 - Agranulocytosis where all leucocytes drop to low levels with fever, ulceration of mouth, rectum, vagina, etc.

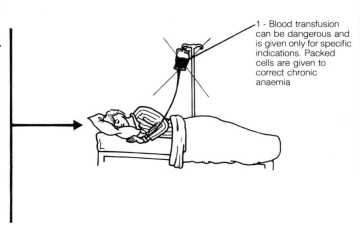

The bone marrow aspirate (or bone trephine) provides cellular material from the red marrow and, as we shall see below, can provide a more certain haematological diagnosis, (by allowing study of the precursor cells), when the peripheral blood film is not diagnostic.

1 - Bone marrow aspirate or bone trephine providing bone marrow for study

2 - The bone marrow provides cellular material for the study of precursor cells

3 - The bone marrow aspirate is done if the peripheral blood film is not diagnostic

BLOOD TRANSFUSION AND THE CROSS-MATCH PROCEDURE

With the modern availability of individual blood products, we should think of a simple blood transfusion as **'red cell therapy'**. However, blood transfusion is a potentially dangerous procedure and should only be performed after careful consideration of the indications. Thus bleeding patients or patients with marrow failure are obvious indications. (Acutely bleeding patients require transfusion with **'whole blood'** whereas transfusion to correct chronic anaemia is usually performed with **'packed cells'**).

1 - Blood transfusion can be dangerous and is given only for specific indications. Packed cells are given to correct chronic anaemia

However, an elderly lady with newly diagnosed pernicious anaemia and an Hb of 6.5g/dl probably does not need a blood transfusion as she is compensated for this and the B_{12} haematinic will correct the anaemia quickly; furthermore, her cardiovascular system is in a high output state and liable to heart failure, due to fluid overload. This proclivity for pulmonary oedema during blood transfusion of anaemic patients is often a problem and a potassium-losing diuretic is often given during the transfusion.

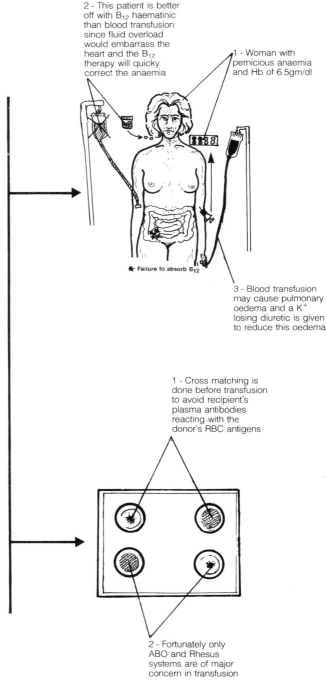

2 - This patient is better off with B_{12} haematinic than blood transfusion since fluid overload would embarrass the heart and the B_{12} therapy will quicky correct the anaemia

1 - Woman with pernicious anaemia and Hb of 6.5gm/dl

★ Failure to absorb B_{12}

3 - Blood transfusion may cause pulmonary oedema and a K^+ losing diuretic is given to reduce this oedema

1 - Cross matching is done before transfusion to avoid recipient's plasma antibodies reacting with the donor's RBC antigens

2 - Fortunately only ABO and Rhesus systems are of major concern in transfusion

Prior to a blood transfusion, a **cross-match** procedure is performed to ensure that the recipient's plasma does not contain **antibodies** which react with the donor's red cell **antigens.** Although all the blood group antigen systems can give rise to transfusion difficulties fortunately only two – the **ABO** and the **Rhesus** systems – are of major importance.

The **ABO** system has four allelomorphic genes: **A₁**, **A₂**, **B** and **O**. The first three genes are responsible for converting a basic substance, **H**, present in all erythrocyte membranes, into **A₁**, **A₂** or **B** antigens. The **O** gene adds nothing to basic **H** – blood group **O**. In the UK, the distribution of the blood groups is:- **Group O**, 46%; **Group A**, 42%; **Group B**, 9%; **Group AB**, 3%. There is a tendency for people to have circulating antibody to the **ABO** antigens that their red cells do not possess, and **anti-A** and **anti-B** are common and important. Because of the presence of these antibodies, it is necessary to transfuse blood with the same **ABO** group as the recipient.

The **Rhesus system** comprises three pairs of allelomorphic genes: **C + c**, **D + d**, **E + e**, where **D** appears to be the most potent antigen and, in the original nomenclature, people with **D** were referred to as **Rhesus positive**. However, other Rhesus antigens and indeed other blood group systems (eg. Kelly, Duffy and Kidd antigenic system) may also prove sufficiently antigenic to provoke a transfusion reaction.

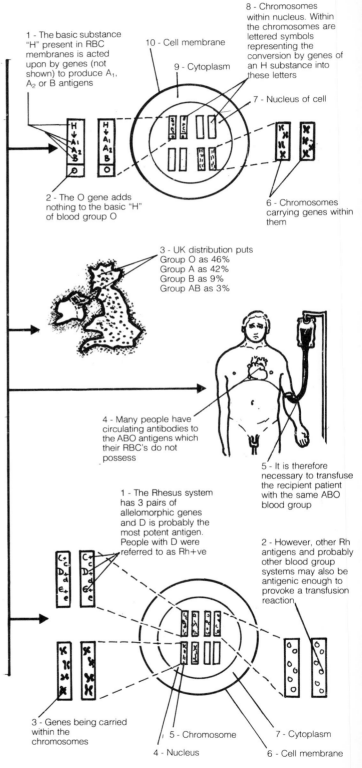

1 - The basic substance "H" present in RBC membranes is acted upon by genes (not shown) to produce A₁, A₂ or B antigens

10 - Cell membrane

9 - Cytoplasm

8 - Chromosomes within nucleus. Within the chromosomes are lettered symbols representing the conversion by genes of an H substance into these letters

7 - Nucleus of cell

2 - The O gene adds nothing to the basic "H" of blood group O

6 - Chromosomes carrying genes within them

3 - UK distribution puts
Group O as 46%
Group A as 42%
Group B as 9%
Group AB as 3%

4 - Many people have circulating antibodies to the ABO antigens which their RBC's do not possess

5 - It is therefore necessary to transfuse the recipient patient with the same ABO blood group

1 - The Rhesus system has 3 pairs of allelomorphic genes and D is probably the most potent antigen. People with D were referred to as Rh+ve

2 - However, other Rh antigens and probably other blood group systems may also be antigenic enough to provoke a transfusion reaction

3 - Genes being carried within the chromosomes

4 - Nucleus

5 - Chromosome

6 - Cell membrane

7 - Cytoplasm

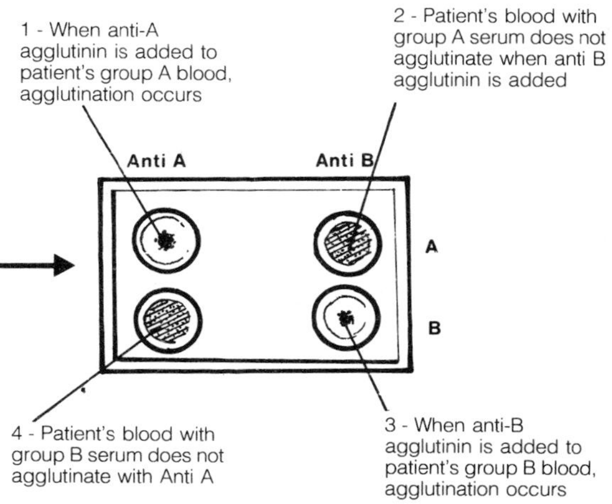

In the cross-match procedure, the **ABO** group is first determined by adding agglutinating **anti-A** and **anti-B** to red cell suspensions from the patient's blood. An agglutinated pellet with **anti-A** but not **anti-B** implies blood group A etc. The Rhesus group may be simply determined by an **anti-D** serum.

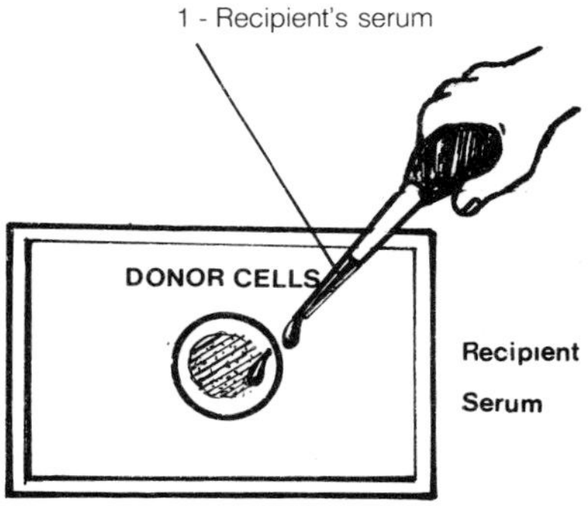

1 - When anti-A agglutinin is added to patient's group A blood, agglutination occurs

2 - Patient's blood with group A serum does not agglutinate when anti B agglutinin is added

Anti A   Anti B

A

B

4 - Patient's blood with group B serum does not agglutinate with Anti A

3 - When anti-B agglutinin is added to patient's group B blood, agglutination occurs

1 - Recipient's serum

DONOR CELLS

Recipient

Serum

The cross-match itself now double checks that there have been no errors in the **ABO** and **Rhesus** typing, and also screens for other potential transfusion reactions. The recipient's serum is added to a suspension of the donor's cells and incubated at 37°C for two hours – the cells are then examined for **agglutination**.

37°C

3 - The cells are then examined for agglutination – a double check for cross matching

2 - The recipient's serum and donor's cells are incubated at 37°C for 2 hours

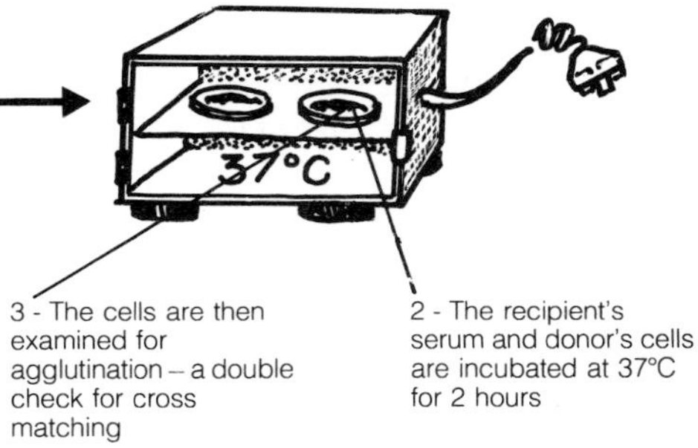

The **Coombs' test,** (the antiglobulin test), should be mentioned at this stage. This test screens for non-agglutinating antibodies in the recipient's serum. The test utilises human **anti-IgG** (or **anti-complement**) and this will cross-link the non-agglutinating antibodies coating donor red cells (in a cross-match suspension) and so bring about visible agglutination.

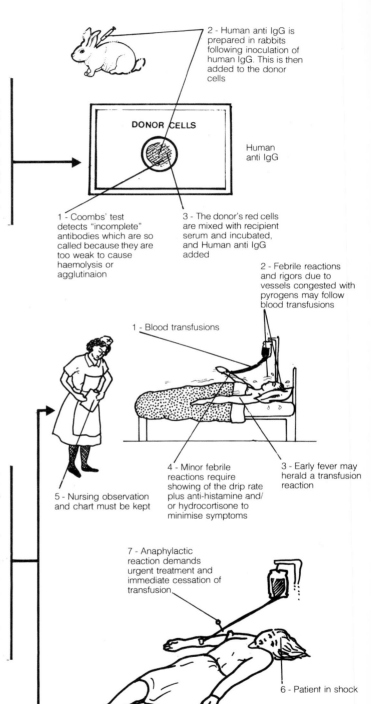

2 - Human anti IgG is prepared in rabbits following inoculation of human IgG. This is then added to the donor cells

DONOR CELLS

Human anti IgG

1 - Coombs' test detects "incomplete" antibodies which are so called because they are too weak to cause haemolysis or agglutinaion

3 - The donor's red cells are mixed with recipient serum and incubated, and Human anti IgG added

2 - Febrile reactions and rigors due to vessels congested with pyrogens may follow blood transfusions

1 - Blood transfusions

4 - Minor febrile reactions require showing of the drip rate plus anti-histamine and/ or hydrocortisone to minimise symptoms

3 - Early fever may herald a transfusion reaction

5 - Nursing observation and chart must be kept

7 - Anaphylactic reaction demands urgent treatment and immediate cessation of transfusion

6 - Patient in shock

UNWANTED SEQUELAE TO BLOOD TRANSFUSION

Simple **febrile reactions** are common with blood transfusions and rigors may occur and may be due to a plethora of pyrogens. However, early fever may also augur a serious transfusion reaction and a frequent and meticulous nursing observation chart must be kept. For minor febrile reactions, an initial slowing of the drip rate together with an antihistamine and/or hydrocortisone may allay symptoms. An anaphylactic reaction demands urgent treatment and immediate cessation of transfusion.

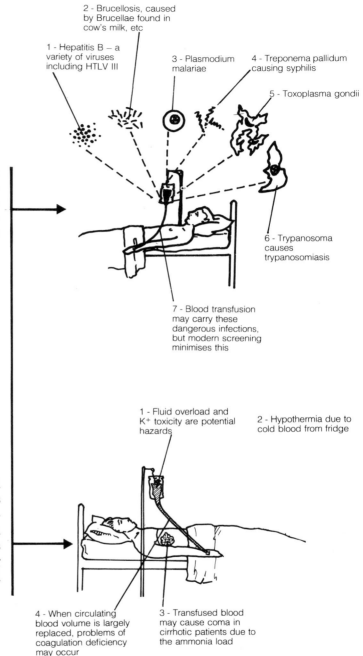

2 - Brucellosis, caused by Brucellae found in cow's milk, etc

1 - Hepatitis B — a variety of viruses including HTLV III

3 - Plasmodium malariae

4 - Treponema pallidum causing syphilis

5 - Toxoplasma gondii

6 - Trypanosoma causes trypanosomiasis

7 - Blood transfusion may carry these dangerous infections, but modern screening minimises this

The potential of transmitting **infections** (eg. malaria, syphilis, toxoplasmosis, trypanosomiasis, brucellosis, hepatitis B, Aids), during blood transfusion must never be forgotten, although with modern screening this should be rare.

1 - Fluid overload and K+ toxicity are potential hazards

2 - Hypothermia due to cold blood from fridge

4 - When circulating blood volume is largely replaced, problems of coagulation deficiency may occur

3 - Transfused blood may cause coma in cirrhotic patients due to the ammonia load

Fluid overload, potassium toxicity and hypothermia are potential hazards as is the precipitation of hepatic coma in cirrhotics, (due to the ammonia load from stored blood). When very large quantities of stored blood are used, the circulating blood volume is largely replaced and coagulation deficiencies may manifest.

MAJOR TRANSFUSION REACTION

With a major **ABO** incompatibility an immediate intravascular haemolytic reaction occurs on initiation of blood transfusion. Facial flushing, rigors, severe loin pain and circulatory collapse may occur, and, if the patient survives this, acute renal failure and extensive haemorrhage (due to defibrination) may both follow. The infusion must be stopped immediately and a mannitol diuresis initiated together with circulatory support.

When blood transfusion is followed by extravascular haemolysis the clinical picture is less acute with chills and perhaps rigors occurring one or more hours after the start of infusion. The most common antibody causing extravascular haemolysis is anti-D. This type of incompatibility is almost never followed by renal failure.

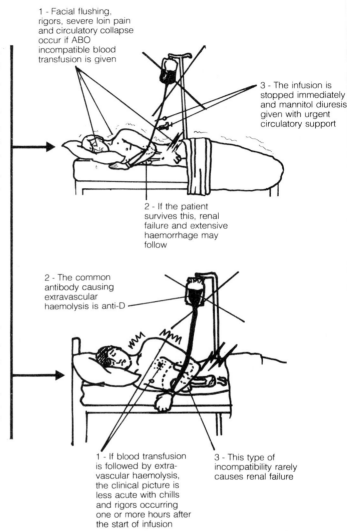

1 - Facial flushing, rigors, severe loin pain and circulatory collapse occur if ABO incompatible blood transfusion is given

3 - The infusion is stopped immediately and mannitol diuresis given with urgent circulatory support

2 - If the patient survives this, renal failure and extensive haemorrhage may follow

2 - The common antibody causing extravascular haemolysis is anti-D

1 - If blood transfusion is followed by extravascular haemolysis, the clinical picture is less acute with chills and rigors occurring one or more hours after the start of infusion

3 - This type of incompatibility rarely causes renal failure

OTHER BLOOD PRODUCTS

Fresh Whole Blood – is useful in hepatic and renal disease and in the newborn – where changes in stored blood are detrimental – eg. increased plasma potassium and ammonia, decreased pH and coagulation factors.

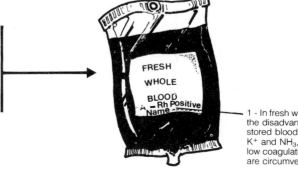

FRESH WHOLE BLOOD – Rh Positive Name

1 - In fresh whole blood, the disadvantages of stored blood (viz. high K^+ and NH_3, low pH, low coagulation factors) are circumvented

Granulocyte Concentrates – Cell separators now exist capable of harvesting large numbers of leucocytes from a donor's blood. A granulocyte transfusion can be life-saving in a septicaemic patient with leukaemia and neutropenia.

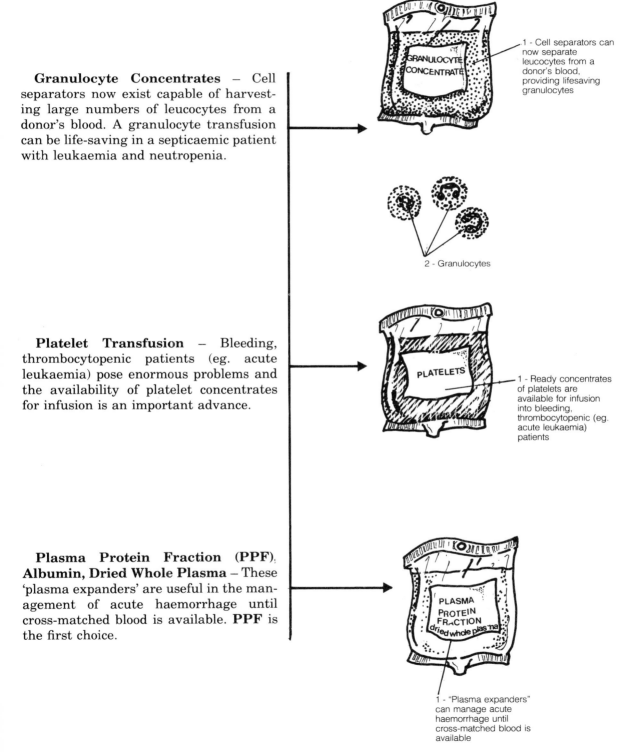

1 - Cell separators can now separate leucocytes from a donor's blood, providing lifesaving granulocytes

2 - Granulocytes

Platelet Transfusion – Bleeding, thrombocytopenic patients (eg. acute leukaemia) pose enormous problems and the availability of platelet concentrates for infusion is an important advance.

1 - Ready concentrates of platelets are available for infusion into bleeding, thrombocytopenic (eg. acute leukaemia) patients

Plasma Protein Fraction (PPF), Albumin, Dried Whole Plasma – These 'plasma expanders' are useful in the management of acute haemorrhage until cross-matched blood is available. **PPF** is the first choice.

1 - "Plasma expanders" can manage acute haemorrhage until cross-matched blood is available

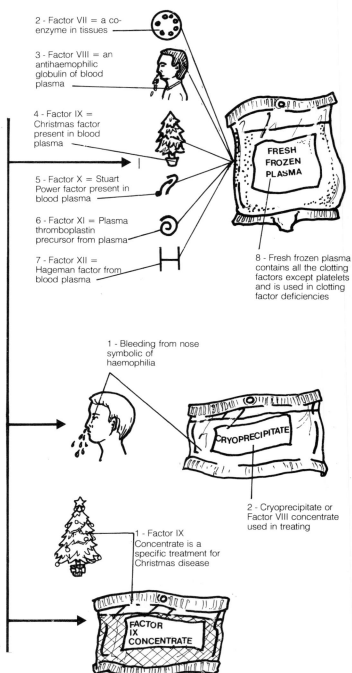

2 - Factor VII = a co-enzyme in tissues

3 - Factor VIII = an antihaemophilic globulin of blood plasma

4 - Factor IX = Christmas factor present in blood plasma

5 - Factor X = Stuart Power factor present in blood plasma

6 - Factor XI = Plasma thromboplastin precursor from plasma

7 - Factor XII = Hageman factor from blood plasma

8 - Fresh frozen plasma contains all the clotting factors except platelets and is used in clotting factor deficiencies

1 - Bleeding from nose symbolic of haemophilia

2 - Cryoprecipitate or Factor VIII concentrate used in treating

1 - Factor IX Concentrate is a specific treatment for Christmas disease

Fresh Frozen Plasma(FFP) – FFP contains all clotting factors except platelets and is used in clotting factor deficiencies unless specific factors are known to be required.

Cryoprecipitate – This is a factor VIII concentrate, derived from FFP, and specific therapy in haemophilia.

Factor IX Concentrate – This concentrate is specific therapy for Christmas disease.

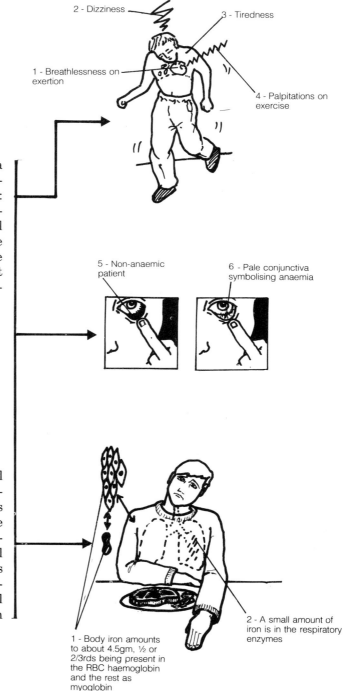

ANAEMIA

The clinical manifestations of anaemia are those of the decreased oxygen carrying capacity of the blood. These are: tiredness, breathlessness on exertion, dizziness, palpitations on exercise, general malaise, insomnia and anorexia. In some elderly patients or those with severe anaemia, heart failure, (often high output failure), occurs or angina pectoris is precipitated.

Iron Deficiency Anaemia – The total body iron of the adult amounts to approximately 4.5g of which half to two thirds is in the erythrocyte haemoglobin and the rest as myogloglobin, storage iron (ferritin, haemosiderin) and a very small amount in respiratory enzymes. There is no physiological mechanism for the excretion of excessive iron and the control seems to be on the absorption. Dietary iron

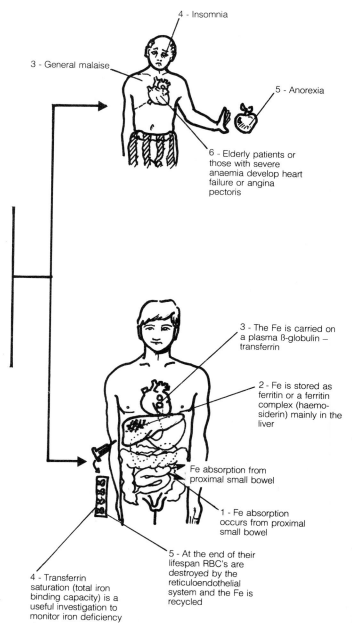

4 - Insomnia

3 - General malaise

5 - Anorexia

6 - Elderly patients or those with severe anaemia develop heart failure or angina pectoris

is absorbed from the proximal small gut and thence carried on a plasma ß globulin – transferrin. The transferrin saturation (**total iron binding** capacity, **TIBC**) is a useful investigation in iron deficiency. Iron is stored as ferritin or the ferritin complex: haemosiderin, largely in the liver. At the end of their life span, erythrocytes are destroyed by the reticuloendothelial system and the iron is recycled.

3 - The Fe is carried on a plasma ß-globulin – transferrin

2 - Fe is stored as ferritin or a ferritin complex (haemosiderin) mainly in the liver

Fe absorption from proximal small bowel

1 - Fe absorption occurs from proximal small bowel

5 - At the end of their lifespan RBC's are destroyed by the reticuloendothelial system and the Fe is recycled

4 - Transferrin saturation (total iron binding capacity) is a useful investigation to monitor iron deficiency

A normal man loses 1–2mg of iron daily which is more than adequately supplied by a good mixed diet. Menstruating women may require an absorption of 3mg per day to remain in balance, and have even larger dietary requirements during pregnancy and lactation.

Dietary deficiency of iron is unusual because meat, eggs and green vegetables all contain good supplies. Malabsorptive causes or iron deficiency are also unusual but are well recognised following gastrectormy, small bowel short circuit procedures in coeliac diseases and other malabsorptive syndromes.

Haemorrhage, particularly chronic bleeding, is the most important cause of iron deficiency anaemia. The gastrointestinal tract is a notorious site for occult bleeding leading to iron deficiency anaemia. There are many causes which include peptic ulcer, hiatus hernia, gastrointestinal tract cancer, ulcerative colitis, parasitic infection, aspirin ingestion. It may be categorically stated that iron deficiency anaemia must always be investigated for its cause and where that cause is occult, the gastro-intestinal tract should be suspected and the stools sent for guaiac testing; Barium studies may be needed.

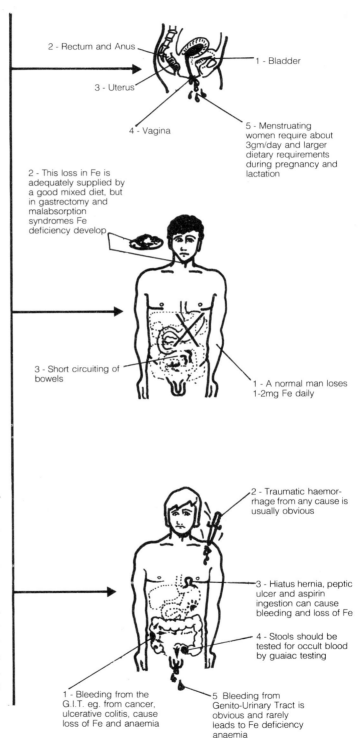

2 - Rectum and Anus

1 - Bladder

3 - Uterus

4 - Vagina

5 - Menstruating women require about 3gm/day and larger dietary requirements during pregnancy and lactation

2 - This loss in Fe is adequately supplied by a good mixed diet, but in gastrectomy and malabsorption syndromes Fe deficiency develop

3 - Short circuiting of bowels

1 - A normal man loses 1-2mg Fe daily

2 - Traumatic haemorrhage from any cause is usually obvious

3 - Hiatus hernia, peptic ulcer and aspirin ingestion can cause bleeding and loss of Fe

4 - Stools should be tested for occult blood by guaiac testing

1 - Bleeding from the G.I.T. eg. from cancer, ulcerative colitis, cause loss of Fe and anaemia

5 Bleeding from Genito-Urinary Tract is obvious and rarely leads to Fe deficiency anaemia

Bleeding from the genito-urinary tract is usually obvious early and does not lead to iron deficiency. Menorrhagia may be accepted by patients and this may then lead to iron deficiency. Traumatic haemorrhage is usually obvious.

6 - Menorrhagia or excessive cyclical bleeding at menstruation can cause Fe deficiency

1 - Increased Fe is required in childhood and adolescence

Increased iron requirements occur in childhood and adolescence and during pregnancy and the puerperium. Iron deficiency in pregnancy is so 'routine' that prophylactic iron supplements are indicated.

2 - Pregnancy demands more Fe

3 - Fe is required in the puerperium

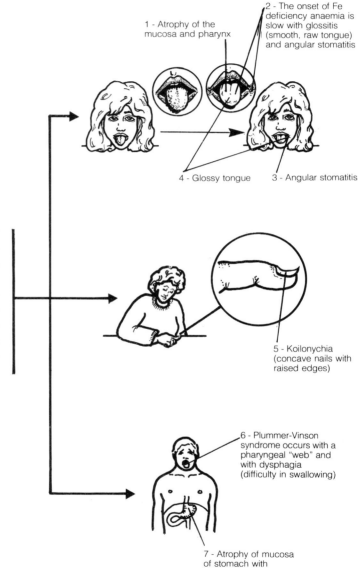

1 - Atrophy of the mucosa and pharynx

2 - The onset of Fe deficiency anaemia is slow with glossitis (smooth, raw tongue) and angular stomatitis

4 - Glossy tongue

3 - Angular stomatitis

5 - Koilonychia (concave nails with raised edges)

6 - Plummer-Vinson syndrome occurs with a pharyngeal "web" and with dysphagia (difficulty in swallowing)

7 - Atrophy of mucosa of stomach with impaired gastric secretion

Clinically, the onset of iron deficiency anaemia is gradual and, in addition to the general symptoms of anaemia, there is often glossitis, (smooth raw tongue), angular stomatitis, koilonychia and atrophy of the mucosa of pharynx and stomach giving rise to dysphagia and impaired gastric secretion. Dysphagia due to a low pharyngeal 'web' may occur — **Plummer-Vinson syndrome**.

The blood indices show an early fall in the **Hb** and **MCV** with, slightly later, a fall in the **MCH** – (a microcytic, hypochromic anaemia). The serum iron is low and the **TIBC** raised. A bone marrow shows no stainable storage iron. **Treatment** is of the underlying disorder (eg. peptic ulcer), but the iron deficiency is nearly always correctable with oral iron. Ferrous sulphate tablets (eg. 200mg oral tds) is inexpensive and satisfactory, although, if gastrointestinal upset occurs, ferrous gluconate is an alternative.

The rise in **Hb** should be at least 2g/dl in 3 weeks following institution of oral iron therapy. Parenteral iron (eg. iron dextran complex, intramuscularly) has few advantages over oral iron except when there is genuine intolerance to oral iron, malabsorption, or the oral formulation is exacerbating gastrointestinal tract disease (eg. ulcerative colitis, peptic ulcer).

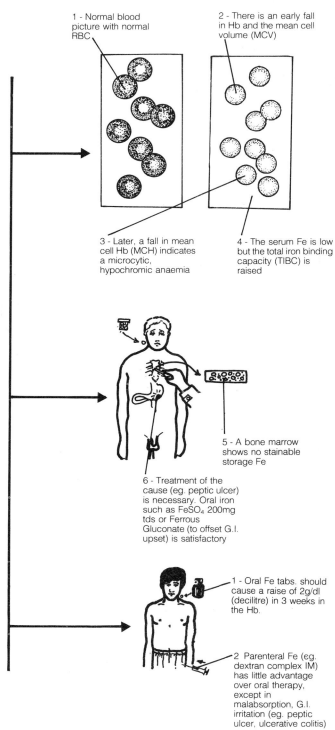

1 - Normal blood picture with normal RBC

2 - There is an early fall in Hb and the mean cell volume (MCV)

3 - Later, a fall in mean cell Hb (MCH) indicates a microcytic, hypochromic anaemia

4 - The serum Fe is low but the total iron binding capacity (TIBC) is raised

5 - A bone marrow shows no stainable storage Fe

6 - Treatment of the cause (eg. peptic ulcer) is necessary. Oral iron such as FeSO$_4$ 200mg tds or Ferrous Gluconate (to offset G.I. upset) is satisfactory

1 - Oral Fe tabs. should cause a raise of 2g/dl (decilitre) in 3 weeks in the Hb.

2 Parenteral Fe (eg. dextran complex IM) has little advantage over oral therapy, except in malabsorption, G.I. irritation (eg. peptic ulcer, ulcerative colitis)

Occasionally, it is necessary to give parenteral iron to replenish stores rapidly (eg. late pregnancy).

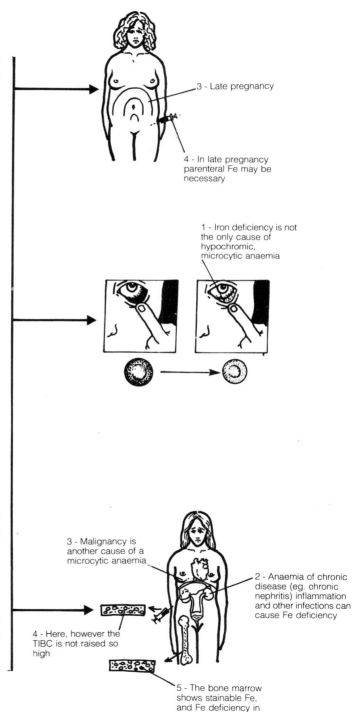

3 - Late pregnancy

4 - In late pregnancy parenteral Fe may be necessary

1 - Iron deficiency is not the only cause of hypochromic, microcytic anaemia

Iron deficiency is not the only cause of a hypochromic, microcytic anaemia. In the so-called 'anaemia of chronic disease' which accompanies chronic inflammation, infection or malignancy, the red cell indices often resemble those of mild iron deficiency except that further investigations do not tend to show a raised **TIBC** and a bone marrow shows stainable iron; the problem appears to be one of iron mobilisation.

3 - Malignancy is another cause of a microcytic anaemia

2 - Anaemia of chronic disease (eg. chronic nephritis) inflammation and other infections can cause Fe deficiency

4 - Here, however the TIBC is not raised so high

5 - The bone marrow shows stainable Fe, and Fe deficiency in these cases is due to failure of Fe mobilization

23

ß thalassaemia minor, (a condition of little clinical importance), often presents a blood picture of a low **MCV** and slightly low **Hb**; an **Hb** electrophoretic strip demonstrating a raised level of **HBA₂** is helpful in diagnosis. In sideroblastic anaemia there is defective porphyrin synthesis to such an extent that iron accumulates in the cytoplasm of the developing red cells, unable to complex with proto-porphyrin. When this iron encrusts mitochondria surrounding a normoblast nucleus, the cell is termed a 'ring sideroblast'. Sideroblastic anaemia may be a hereditary trait or a primary acquired condition in the elderly. Other causes are: lead poisoning, alcohol excess, pyridoxine deficiency or other marrow disease (eg. acute leukaemia). Many cases of sideroblastic anaemia are associated with a microcytic picture; treatment is of any underlying cause. Pyridoxine and folic acid supplements may help.

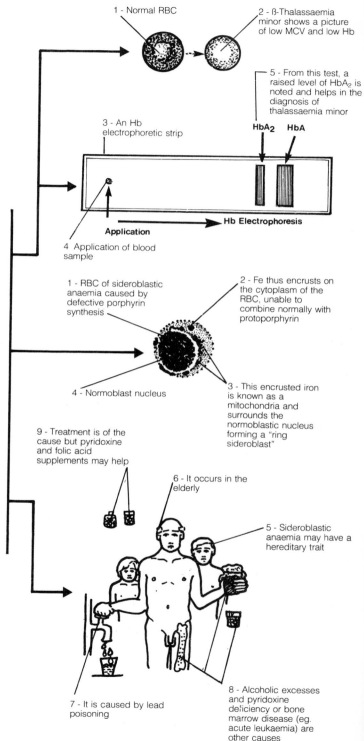

1 - Normal RBC

2 - ß-Thalassaemia minor shows a picture of low MCV and low Hb

5 - From this test, a raised level of HbA₂ is noted and helps in the diagnosis of thalassaemia minor

3 - An Hb electrophoretic strip

HbA₂   HbA

Hb Electrophoresis

Application

4 Application of blood sample

1 - RBC of sideroblastic anaemia caused by defective porphyrin synthesis

2 - Fe thus encrusts on the cytoplasm of the RBC, unable to combine normally with protoporphyrin

3 - This encrusted iron is known as a mitochondria and surrounds the normoblastic nucleus forming a "ring sideroblast"

4 - Normoblast nucleus

9 - Treatment is of the cause but pyridoxine and folic acid supplements may help

6 - It occurs in the elderly

5 - Sideroblastic anaemia may have a hereditary trait

7 - It is caused by lead poisoning

8 - Alcoholic excesses and pyridoxine deficiency or bone marrow disease (eg. acute leukaemia) are other causes

Megaloblastic Anaemia – In mega-loblastic anaemia, there are large red blood cells circulating in the peripheral blood (macrocytes: **MCV** more than 96 fl) and in the bone marrow the abnormally large erythroid precursor cells have nuc-lei too large and immature for their stage of development and haemoglobinisation of the cytoplasm – (megaloblasts). In addition, the marrow tends to be hyper-plastic due to ineffective erythopoiesis, (that is, many megaloblasts fail to mature and die in the marrow).

This high red cell turnover leads to a slightly elevated plasma bilirubin and high lactate dehydrogenase levels. There is often an associated mild leucopenia and thrombocytopenia with giant metamyelo-cytes in the marrow and hypersegmented neutrophils in the peripheral blood.

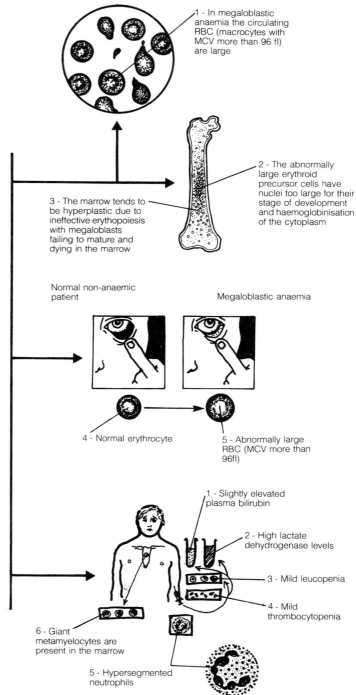

1 - In megaloblastic anaemia the circulating RBC (macrocytes with MCV more than 96 fl) are large

2 - The abnormally large erythroid precursor cells have nuclei too large for their stage of development and haemoglobinisation of the cytoplasm

3 - The marrow tends to be hyperplastic due to ineffective erythopoiesis with megaloblasts failing to mature and dying in the marrow

Normal non-anaemic patient

Megaloblastic anaemia

4 - Normal erythrocyte

5 - Abnormally large RBC (MCV more than 96fl)

1 - Slightly elevated plasma bilirubin

2 - High lactate dehydrogenase levels

3 - Mild leucopenia

4 - Mild thrombocytopenia

6 - Giant metamyelocytes are present in the marrow

5 - Hypersegmented neutrophils

There are two common causes of megaloblastic anaemia: vitamin B_{12} deficiency and folic acid deficiency, and several extremely rare causes eg. **Lesch-Nyan syndrome**, vitamin E deficiency, sideroblastic anaemia, erythroleukaemia.

Vitamin B_{12}, a cobalamin, contains a cobalt containing corrin ring linked to a nucleotide; it is present in animals and bacteria but not in plants. Ingested B_{12} is absorbed from the distal ileum following complexing with a specific glycoprotein secreted by the gastic parietal cells, (intrinsic factor, **IF**). Absorbed B_{12} is carried in the plasma on carrier proteins (transcobalamins) and stored in the liver; normal liver contains several years' reserve of B_{12}.

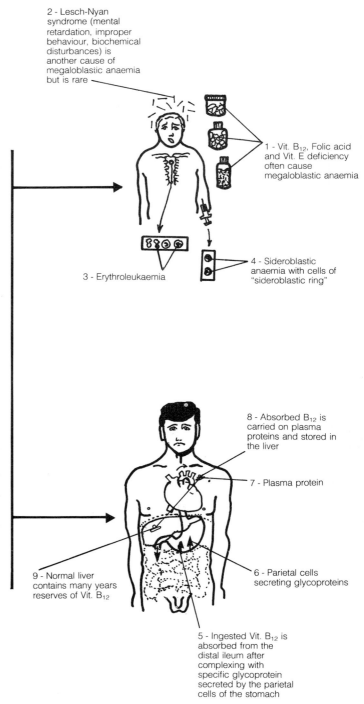

2 - Lesch-Nyan syndrome (mental retardation, improper behaviour, biochemical disturbances) is another cause of megaloblastic anaemia but is rare

1 - Vit. B_{12}, Folic acid and Vit. E deficiency often cause megaloblastic anaemia

3 - Erythroleukaemia

4 - Sideroblastic anaemia with cells of "sideroblastic ring"

8 - Absorbed B_{12} is carried on plasma proteins and stored in the liver

7 - Plasma protein

6 - Parietal cells secreting glycoproteins

9 - Normal liver contains many years reserves of Vit. B_{12}

5 - Ingested Vit. B_{12} is absorbed from the distal ileum after complexing with specific glycoprotein secreted by the parietal cells of the stomach

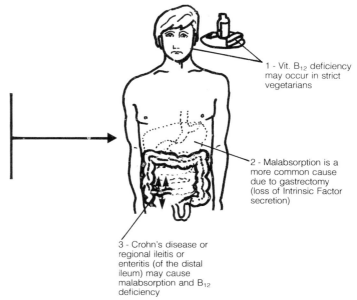

Vitamin B_{12} deficiency is occasionally due to dietary deficiency in strict vegetarians but usually the cause is malabsorption: eg. postgastrectomy (no **IF** secretion), pernicious anaemia, distal small bowel disease (eg. Crohn's disease).

1 - Vit. B_{12} deficiency may occur in strict vegetarians

2 - Malabsorption is a more common cause due to gastrectomy (loss of Intrinsic Factor secretion)

3 - Crohn's disease or regional ileitis or enteritis (of the distal ileum) may cause malabsorption and B_{12} deficiency

1 - Pernicious anaemia is a disease of the elderly, commoner in women, with a familial tendency and associated with auto-immune disorders

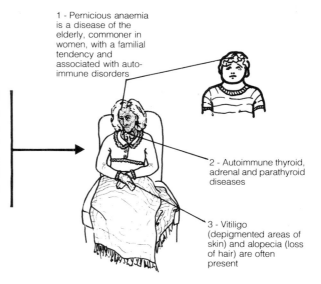

Pernicious Anaemia – Pernicious Anaemia (**PA**) is a disease of the elderly, being more common in women, with a slight familial tendency and an association with other auto-immune disorders, (notably auto-immune thyroid, adrenal and parathyroid disease) and with vitiligo and alopecia.

2 - Autoimmune thyroid, adrenal and parathyroid diseases

3 - Vitiligo (depigmented areas of skin) and alopecia (loss of hair) are often present

In **PA** there is an immune reaction against the gastric parietal cells and parietal cell auto-antibodies, and auto-antibodies to **IF** itself are demonstrable in the sera of most patients. The consequences are gastric achlorhydria and absent **IF** secretion, with failure to absorb B_{12}. The clinical onset is very insidious and frequently patients present with very low **Hb** values. In addition to their pallor, mild jaundice may just be detectable clinically, and a smooth sore tongue may also be noted; diarrhoea and dyspepsia are common. Mild splenomegaly may occur. Very frequently, the patients complain of numbness or tingling in the fingers and toes; much less frequently there are signs of impairment of neurological functions subserved by the posterior and lateral columns of the spinal cord. This unusual neurological complication of B_{12} deficiency is called **subacute combined degeneration of the cord.**

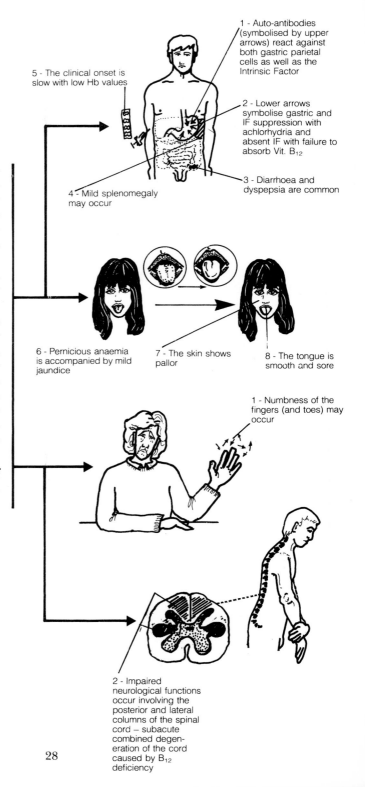

1 - Auto-antibodies (symbolised by upper arrows) react against both gastric parietal cells as well as the Intrinsic Factor

2 - Lower arrows symbolise gastric and IF suppression with achlorhydria and absent IF with failure to absorb Vit. B_{12}

3 - Diarrhoea and dyspepsia are common

4 - Mild splenomegaly may occur

5 - The clinical onset is slow with low Hb values

6 - Pernicious anaemia is accompanied by mild jaundice

7 - The skin shows pallor

8 - The tongue is smooth and sore

1 - Numbness of the fingers (and toes) may occur

2 - Impaired neurological functions occur involving the posterior and lateral columns of the spinal cord – subacute combined degeneration of the cord caused by B_{12} deficiency

A low serum B_{12} level is essential for the diagnosis of B_{12} deficiency, but a low B_{12} level may also occur in other conditions, (including folate deficiency). The diagnosis of **PA** is confirmed by a **Schilling test**, but this test may be delayed until treatment is commenced: The subject is first given a large intramuscular dose of B_{12} to saturate tissue-binding sites. Oral doses of radioactively labelled B_{12} are then given without and later with intrinsic factor. Radioactive B_{12} excretion in the urine is monitored and only when the oral dose is accompanied by **IF** will the urinary excretion of the labelled vitamin be significant in **PA** patients.

Treatment of **PA** is best achieved by at least six intramuscular injections of hydroxocobalamin (1000mg). These are given over a three week period at intervals of approximately 3 days. Blood transfusion is avoided unless the patient is extremely anaemic when slow transfusions of packed cells (250–500ml) are carefully performed. The haematological response to

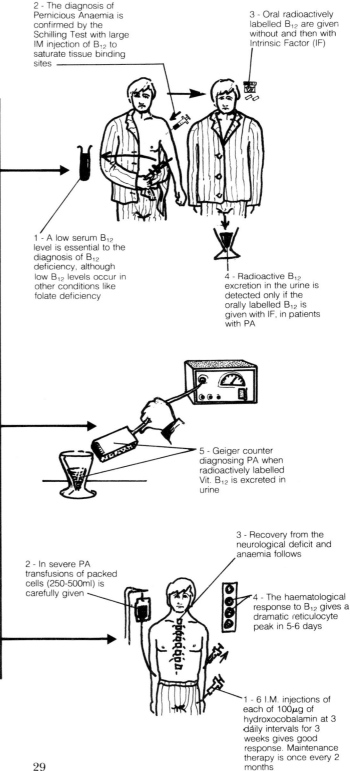

2 - The diagnosis of Pernicious Anaemia is confirmed by the Schilling Test with large IM injection of B_{12} to saturate tissue binding sites

3 - Oral radioactively labelled B_{12} are given without and then with Intrinsic Factor (IF)

1 - A low serum B_{12} level is essential to the diagnosis of B_{12} deficiency, although low B_{12} levels occur in other conditions like folate deficiency

4 - Radioactive B_{12} excretion in the urine is detected only if the orally labelled B_{12} is given with IF, in patients with PA

5 - Geiger counter diagnosing PA when radioactively labelled Vit. B_{12} is excreted in urine

3 - Recovery from the neurological deficit and anaemia follows

2 - In severe PA transfusions of packed cells (250-500ml) is carefully given

4 - The haematological response to B_{12} gives a dramatic reticulocyte peak in 5-6 days

1 - 6 I.M. injections of each of 100μg of hydroxocobalamin at 3 daily intervals for 3 weeks gives good response. Maintenance therapy is once every 2 months

B$_{12}$ is dramatic with a reticulocyte peak at 5–6 days and thereafter recovery from the anaemia and some recovery of neurological deficit. Maintenance **B$_{12}$** therapy of intramuscular hydroxocobalamin (1000mg) once every two months is satisfactory for all patients.

There is a slightly increased risk of gastric carcinoma in patients with **PA**.

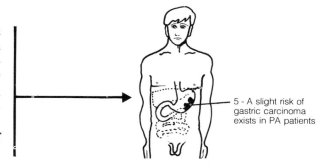

5 - A slight risk of gastric carcinoma exists in PA patients

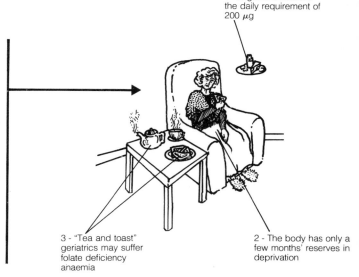

1 - A good diet offers the daily requirement of 200 μg

Folic Acid Deficiency – Folic acid is a pteroylglutamate that is a co-factor in one carbon transfer, essential to **DNA** synthesis. Folic acid is found in many foodstuffs particularly fresh leafy vegetables and fruit. The daily requirements are approximately 200 μg and are easily met by a good diet; the body's reserves are enough for a few months of deprivation. Dietary folate deficiency is one possible cause of folate deficiency anaemia (eg."the tea and toast geriatric"), but so too are the increased bodily requirements for folic acid in, for example, pregnancy, early childhood, conditions of high cell proliferation

3 - "Tea and toast" geriatrics may suffer folate deficiency anaemia

2 - The body has only a few months' reserves in deprivation

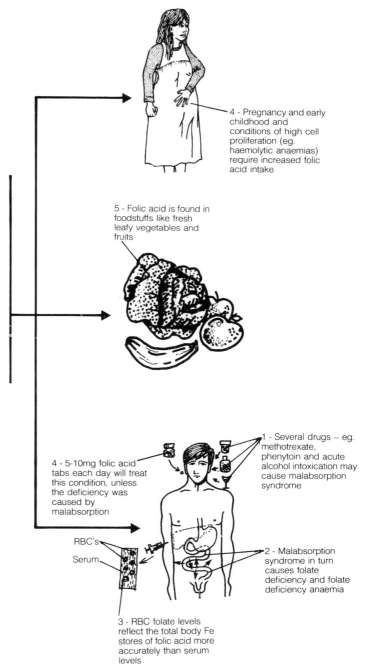

4 - Pregnancy and early childhood and conditions of high cell proliferation (eg. haemolytic anaemias) require increased folic acid intake

5 - Folic acid is found in foodstuffs like fresh leafy vegetables and fruits

1 - Several drugs – eg. methotrexate, phenytoin and acute alcohol intoxication may cause malabsorption syndrome

4 - 5-10mg folic acid tabs each day will treat this condition, unless the deficiency was caused by malabsorption

2 - Malabsorption syndrome in turn causes folate deficiency and folate deficiency anaemia

RBC's

Serum

3 - RBC folate levels reflect the total body Fe stores of folic acid more accurately than serum levels

(eg. haemolytic anaemia). Folate supplements are indicated in all chronic haemolytic anaemias. Malabsorption states can cause folate deficiency and several drugs are well-recognised to interfere with folate metabolism (eg. methotrexate, phenytoin, acute alcohol intoxication). Red cell folate levels more accurately reflect total body stores of folic acid than serum levels and the diagnosis of folate deficiency megaloblastic anaemia should be based on this test. Unless malabsorption is the primary problem, oral folic acid (5–10mg/day) is the treatment of choice.

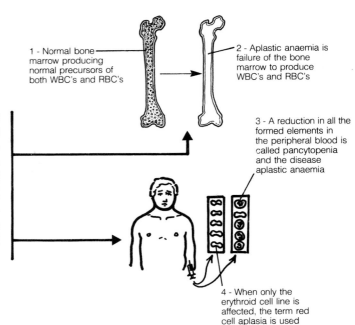

1 - Bone marrow

2 - Some anaemias have a high MCV value but with no evidence of megaloblastosis in the bone marrow

3 - Chronic alcoholism and liver disease are two causes of this condition with reticulocytosis (immature RBC's without network of granules)

The MCV is raised in anaemia in these conditions and also in aplastic, haemolytic and leucoerythroblastic anaemia

4 - The MCV is raised in haemolytic anaemia

5 - Aplastic anaemia is failure of the bone marrow to produce RBC's

6 - MCV is also raised in leucoerythroblastic conditions

Macrocytic, Non-Megaloblastic Anaemia – There are certain conditions which give rise to an anaemia with a very high **MCV** value but there is no evidence of megaloblastosis in the bone marrow. Chronic alcoholism and liver disease are two well-recognised causes and a reticulocytosis due to any cause will tend to raise the **MCV**, ('shift macrocytes'). The **MCV** may also be raised in anaemias of primarily aplastic, haemolytic or leucoerythroblastic origin.

1 - Normal bone marrow producing normal precursors of both WBC's and RBC's

2 - Aplastic anaemia is failure of the bone marrow to produce WBC's and RBC's

3 - A reduction in all the formed elements in the peripheral blood is called pancytopenia and the disease aplastic anaemia

Aplastic Anaemia – Failure of the bone marrow to produce one or more of its cell lines results in anaemia, thrombocytopenia or leucopenia (particularly neutropenia). When there is a reduction in all the formed elements in the peripheral blood (pancytopenia), the disease is referred to as aplastic anaemia; when only the erythroid cell line is affected the term red cell aplasia is used.

4 - When only the erythroid cell line is affected, the term red cell aplasia is used

In some cases of aplastic anaemia, no cause can be found, (idiopathic aplastic anaemia). In other cases the disease may be congenital or familial and be associated with skeletal growth anomalies (**Fanconi's anaemia**). In other cases, marrow aplasia occurs secondary to toxic insults such as irradiation and drugs. With regard to drugs, there are dose-related marrow aplasias, (eg. with cytotoxic alkylating agents) and the idiosyncratic drug reactions such as rarely occur with chloramphenicol, phenylbutazone, gold and tolbutamide.

Acute transient aplastic marrow episodes may occur in acute infections (especially viral infections) and during the course of some haemolytic anaemias (eg. aplastic crisis in sickle cell anaemia). Malignant conditions infiltrating marrow may simulate aplastic anaemia. It should also be noted that a less serious, hypoplastic marrow may occur in hypopituitarism, myxoedema, Addison's disease and uraemia.

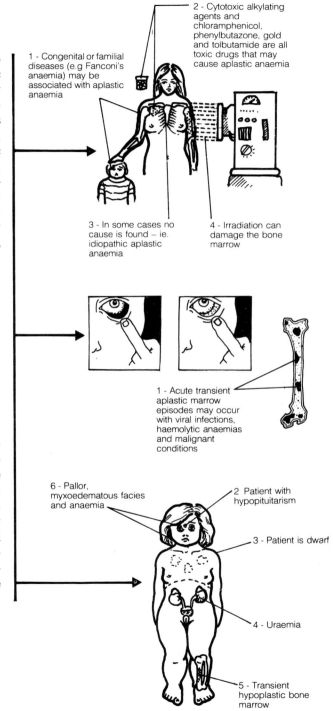

1 - Congenital or familial diseases (e.g Fanconi's anaemia) may be associated with aplastic anaemia

2 - Cytotoxic alkylating agents and chloramphenicol, phenylbutazone, gold and tolbutamide are all toxic drugs that may cause aplastic anaemia

3 - In some cases no cause is found – ie. idiopathic aplastic anaemia

4 - Irradiation can damage the bone marrow

1 - Acute transient aplastic marrow episodes may occur with viral infections, haemolytic anaemias and malignant conditions

6 - Pallor, myxoedematous facies and anaemia

2 Patient with hypopituitarism

3 - Patient is dwarf

4 - Uraemia

5 - Transient hypoplastic bone marrow

The **clinical features** relate to the severity of the anaemia, thrombocytopenia and neutropenia. However, thrombocytopenia is usually pronounced and bleeding tendencies are common, (ecchymosis, purpura, retinal and cerebral haemorrhages). The peripheral blood count shows pancytopenia of variable degree and the bone marrow is hypocellular. In some patients, the disease is explosive with rapid deterioration and death a few

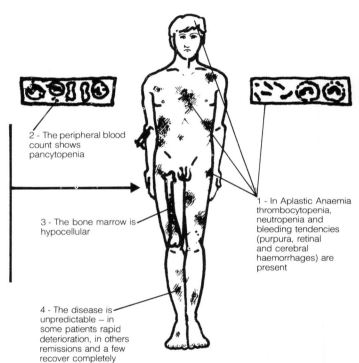

2 - The peripheral blood count shows pancytopenia

3 - The bone marrow is hypocellular

4 - The disease is unpredictable — in some patients rapid deterioration, in others remissions and a few recover completely

1 - In Aplastic Anaemia thrombocytopenia, neutropenia and bleeding tendencies (purpura, retinal and cerebral haemorrhages) are present

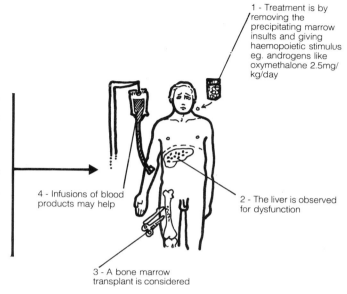

1 - Treatment is by removing the precipitating marrow insults and giving haemopoietic stimulus eg. androgens like oxymethalone 2.5mg/kg/day

4 - Infusions of blood products may help

2 - The liver is observed for dysfunction

3 - A bone marrow transplant is considered

weeks after onset. In others, it may be long lasting but with remissions followed by fatal relapse or occasionally by complete recovery. **Treatment** involves removal of any precipitating marrow insult, haematological support with infusions of blood products, a haemopoietic stimulus (usually androgens eg. oxymethalone 2.5mg/kg/day – watching for hepatic dysfunction), and the consideration of a bone marrow transplant at a specialist centre.

Red Cell Aplasia – Pure red cell aplasia is characterised by an anaemia which is normocytic, (or occasionally macrocytic), and normochromic and associated with bone marrow erythroid hypoplasia. The myeloid and platelet series are normal. Various drugs (eg. chloramphericol, sulphonamides) may cause this condition but there is a well recognised association with thymoma which may be of immunologic basis. Other cases are idiopathic.

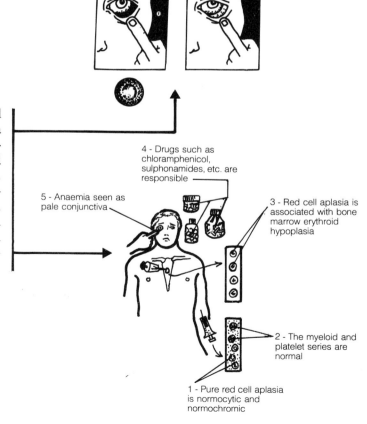

4 - Drugs such as chloramphenicol, sulphonamides, etc. are responsible

5 - Anaemia seen as pale conjunctiva

3 - Red cell aplasia is associated with bone marrow erythroid hypoplasia

2 - The myeloid and platelet series are normal

1 - Pure red cell aplasia is normocytic and normochromic

Agranulocytosis – Here there is a profound deficiency of circulating blood granulocytes and the virtual absence of neutrophils renders the patient very susceptible to overwhelming septicaemic infection. The most important causes to recognise are drugs (eg. phenylbutazone, phenothiazines, sulphonamides, antithyroid drugs etc.). Any possible precipitating agents must be immediately withdrawn and any infection treated with intravenous, combination antibiotic therapy with or without granulocyte infusions. The period of agranulocytosis is usually self-limiting.

HAEMOLYTIC ANAEMIA

The normal life span of the peripheral blood erythrocyte is approximately 120 days. A haemolytic state may be defined as a condition in which the mature erythrocyte is destroyed prematurely. However, the haemolytic state does not always lead to an anaemia as the normal marrow can often compensate for a severalfold increase in red cell destruction.

Patients with haemolytic anaemia usually have a normochromic, normocytic anaemia although it may appear macrocytic when the reticulocyte count is high or be microcytic in thalassaemia.

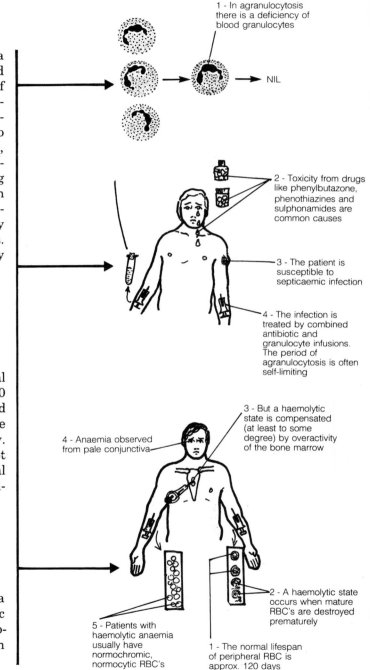

1 - In agranulocytosis there is a deficiency of blood granulocytes

NIL

2 - Toxicity from drugs like phenylbutazone, phenothiazines and sulphonamides are common causes

3 - The patient is susceptible to septicaemic infection

4 - The infection is treated by combined antibiotic and granulocyte infusions. The period of agranulocytosis is often self-limiting

3 - But a haemolytic state is compensated (at least to some degree) by overactivity of the bone marrow

4 - Anaemia observed from pale conjunctiva

2 - A haemolytic state occurs when mature RBC's are destroyed prematurely

5 - Patients with haemolytic anaemia usually have normochromic, normocytic RBC's

1 - The normal lifespan of peripheral RBC is approx. 120 days

The blood smear shows polychromasia of the red cells, (the counterpart of special staining for reticulocytes), and the red cell morphology may be pathognomonic of the underlying disease (see below). The reticulocyte count is high, perhaps 40% of the total red cell count; (one should always relate the percentage reticulocyte count to the total red cell count). The bone marrow is hyperplastic and the red cell precursor cells dominate (erythroid-hyperplasia); the normal myeloid:erythroid ratio of 4:1 is reversed.

The increased red cell destruction leads to an elevation of the serum unconjugated bilirubin and raised urinary urobilinogen, (but not urinary bilirubin – hence the term: acholuric jaundice). An increased incidence of pigment gall stones is present in all chronic haemolytic anaemias. When there is severe intravascular haemolysis, haemoglobinaemia, methaemoglobinaemia and haemoglobinuria occur; more commonly the serum levels of the free carrier protein: haptoglobin are found to be low, due to complexing with released haemoglobin.

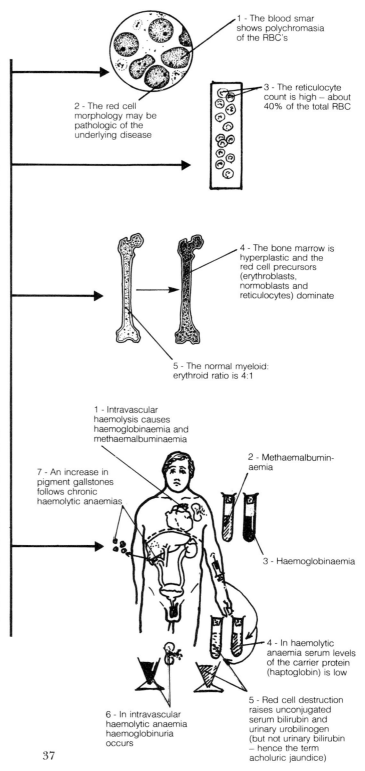

1 - The blood smar shows polychromasia of the RBC's

2 - The red cell morphology may be pathologic of the underlying disease

3 - The reticulocyte count is high – about 40% of the total RBC

4 - The bone marrow is hyperplastic and the red cell precursors (erythroblasts, normoblasts and reticulocytes) dominate

5 - The normal myeloid:erythroid ratio is 4:1

1 - Intravascular haemolysis causes haemoglobinaemia and methaemalbuminaemia

7 - An increase in pigment gallstones follows chronic haemolytic anaemias

2 - Methaemalbumin-aemia

3 - Haemoglobinaemia

4 - In haemolytic anaemia serum levels of the carrier protein (haptoglobin) is low

5 - Red cell destruction raises unconjugated serum bilirubin and urinary urobilinogen (but not urinary bilirubin – hence the term acholuric jaundice)

6 - In intravascular haemolytic anaemia haemoglobinuria occurs

In general terms, the causes of haemolytic anaemia may be divided into:-

1 Intrinsic disorders of the red cell

a) **Of the membrane** – eg. hereditary spherocytosis, hereditary elliptocytosis, paroxysmal nocturnal haemoglobinuria etc.

b) **Of the enzymes** – eg. glucose – 6 phosphate dehydrogenase deficiency, pyrurate kinase deficiency etc.

c) **Of haemoglobin (haemoglobinopathies)** – eg. sickle cell anaemia, thalassaemia.

2 Extrinsic disorders affecting the red cell

a) **Those with antibody production**

b) **Those without antibody production**

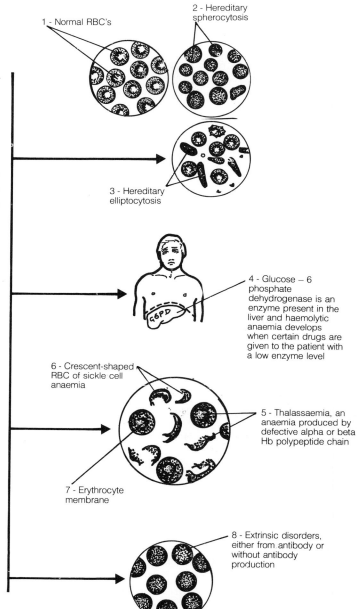

1 - Normal RBC's

2 - Hereditary spherocytosis

3 - Hereditary elliptocytosis

4 - Glucose – 6 phosphate dehydrogenase is an enzyme present in the liver and haemolytic anaemia develops when certain drugs are given to the patient with a low enzyme level

6 - Crescent-shaped RBC of sickle cell anaemia

5 - Thalassaemia, an anaemia produced by defective alpha or beta Hb polypeptide chain

7 - Erythrocyte membrane

8 - Extrinsic disorders, either from antibody or without antibody production

Hereditary Spherocytosis – This rare autosomal dominant disease is associated with small round red cells (**spherocytes**) of reduced life expectancy due to premature destruction in the spleen. The clinical picture is of mild (acholuric) jaundice in an otherwise fit child. Other more severely affected children may be more severely anaemic or sustain transient 'aplastic crises'. The spleen is often enlarged and its removal is the most effective form of therapy. There is no specific therapy for the underlying erythrocyte membrane defect.

Paroxysmal Nocturnal Haemoglobinuria (PNH)

This rare form of acquired haemolytic anaemia is associated with leucopenia and thrombocytopenia and tends to affect people in the 3rd – 4th decades of life. The underlying defect seems to be an increased sensitivity to the lytic effects of complement. The major clinical features are acute episodes of intravascular haemolysis (often nocturnal) with haemoglobinuria, more chronic haemolysis, thrombotic episodes (which may be fatal) and aplastic marrow crises. **Treatment** is supportive care, with transfusions of washed cells.

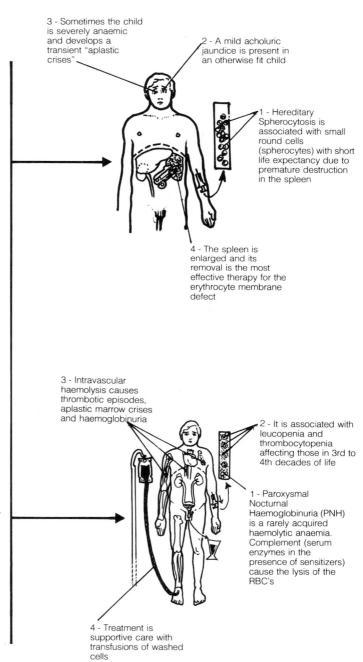

3 - Sometimes the child is severely anaemic and develops a transient "aplastic crises"

2 - A mild acholuric jaundice is present in an otherwise fit child

1 - Hereditary Spherocytosis is associated with small round cells (spherocytes) with short life expectancy due to premature destruction in the spleen

4 - The spleen is enlarged and its removal is the most effective therapy for the erythrocyte membrane defect

3 - Intravascular haemolysis causes thrombotic episodes, aplastic marrow crises and haemoglobinuria

2 - It is associated with leucopenia and thrombocytopenia affecting those in 3rd to 4th decades of life

1 - Paroxysmal Nocturnal Haemoglobinuria (PNH) is a rarely acquired haemolytic anaemia. Complement (serum enzymes in the presence of sensitizers) cause the lysis of the RBC's

4 - Treatment is supportive care with transfusions of washed cells

Glucose 6-phosphate dehydrogenase (G6PD) deficiency – The gene for **G6PD** is located on the **X chromosome** and thus this enzymopathy is inherited as a sex-linked recessive, manifesting almost exclusively in males. Although there are at least three mutant variants of **G6PD**, (African, Mediterranean and Caucasian), the most important **G6PD** deiciency is that which is found in African races.

Patients are usually symptomless unless exposed to oxidants. **G6PD** is important in the maintenance of haemoglobin iron in the reduced ferrous states; in the presence of oxidants, the **G6PD** deficit is unmasked. Oxidants include antimalarials (eg. primaquine), sulphonamides, streptomycin, isoniazid, aspirin, phenytoin etc. The anaemia commences within a few days of taking the oxidant drug and is of variable severity. Severe haemolytic anaemia with rigors and haemoglobinuria may occur. The blood film may show denatured **Hb** in the red cells (**Heinz bodies**). Fortunately, the attacks are self-limiting.

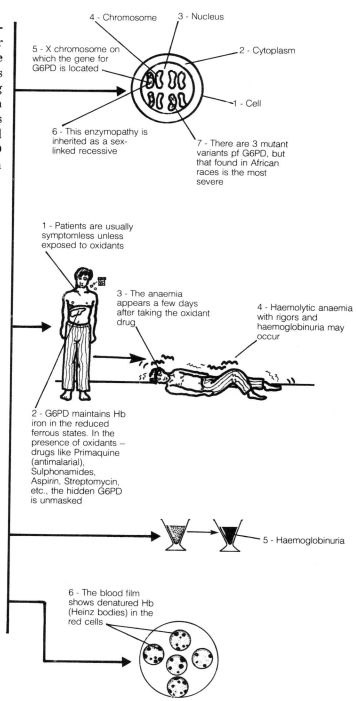

4 - Chromosome

3 - Nucleus

5 - X chromosome on which the gene for G6PD is located

2 - Cytoplasm

1 - Cell

6 - This enzymopathy is inherited as a sex-linked recessive

7 - There are 3 mutant variants pf G6PD, but that found in African races is the most severe

1 - Patients are usually symptomless unless exposed to oxidants

3 - The anaemia appears a few days after taking the oxidant drug

4 - Haemolytic anaemia with rigors and haemoglobinuria may occur

2 - G6PD maintains Hb iron in the reduced ferrous states. In the presence of oxidants – drugs like Primaquine (antimalarial), Sulphonamides, Aspirin, Streptomycin, etc., the hidden G6PD is unmasked

5 - Haemoglobinuria

6 - The blood film shows denatured Hb (Heinz bodies) in the red cells

The Haemoglobinopathies

Haemoglobinopathies are inherited disorders of globin synthesis. They comprise firstly the thalassaemias in which the synthesis of globin chains is impaired (eg. defective ß chain synthesis in ß thalassaemia) and secondly the abnormal haemoglobin syndromes in which there are amino acid variants in the peptide chain sequence (eg. sickle cell disease).

ß Thalassaemia Minor – This heterozygous state is a relatively benign condition. The patient has a mild microcytic anaemia and raised **Hb A$_2$** and **Hb F** levels.

ß Thalassaemia Major – This is the homozygous state and there is grossly defective synthesis of adult haemoglobin (**Hb A**) but this takes until about 6 months of age to manifest clinically.

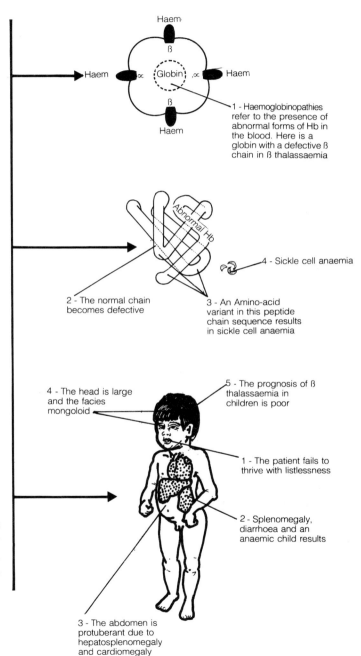

1 - Haemoglobinopathies refer to the presence of abnormal forms of Hb in the blood. Here is a globin with a defective ß chain in ß thalassaemia

2 - The normal chain becomes defective

3 - An Amino-acid variant in this peptide chain sequence results in sickle cell anaemia

4 - Sickle cell anaemia

4 - The head is large and the facies mongoloid

5 - The prognosis of ß thalassaemia in children is poor

1 - The patient fails to thrive with listlessness

2 - Splenomegaly, diarrhoea and an anaemic child results

3 - The abdomen is protuberant due to hepatosplenomegaly and cardiomegaly

Failure to thrive, listlessness, diarrhoea, splenomegaly occuring in an anaemic child with a large head and mongoloid facies suggest the diagnosis. The abdomen is usually protuberant due to hepatosplenomegaly, and cardiomegaly is also common.

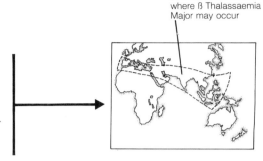

6 - Area in the world where ß Thalassaemia Major may occur

Bone marrow hyperplasia produces osteoporosis – thinned bone cortices with radiologically apparent trabeculae are very characteristic in the hands and skull (hair on end appearance). The blood picture shows a microcytic, hypochromic anaemia and the haemoglobin is mainly foetal (Hb F). There is a reticulocytosis and targeting of red cells is characteristic.

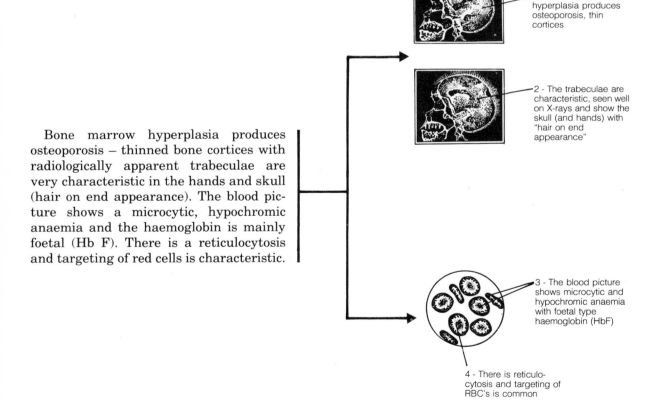

1 - Bone marrow hyperplasia produces osteoporosis, thin cortices

2 - The trabeculae are characteristic, seen well on X-rays and show the skull (and hands) with "hair on end appearance"

3 - The blood picture shows microcytic and hypochromic anaemia with foetal type haemoglobin (HbF)

4 - There is reticulocytosis and targeting of RBC's is common

The outlook in ß thalassaemia major is poor, the children being feeble, prone to infection and anaemia, and requiring transfusions. Many die before puberty due to infection. In those surviving, iron overload (from multiple transfusions) may lead to heart failure.

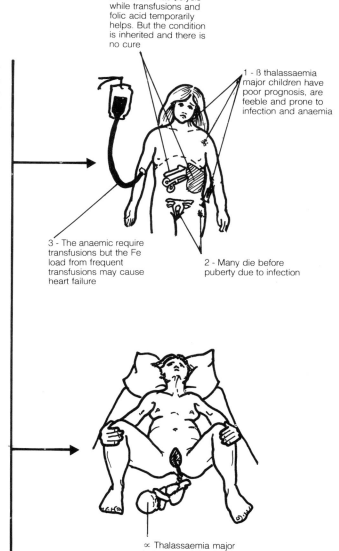

4 - Splenectomy may benefit the haemolysis while transfusions and folic acid temporarily helps. But the condition is inherited and there is no cure

1 - ß thalassaemia major children have poor prognosis, are feeble and prone to infection and anaemia

3 - The anaemic require transfusions but the Fe load from frequent transfusions may cause heart failure

2 - Many die before puberty due to infection

The condition is inherited and there is no cure. Transfusions are required to maintain reasonable health. Splenectomy may be beneficial when haemolysis is great. Folic acid deficiency should be corrected.

∝ **Thalassaemia** – ∝ thalassaemia major is incompatible with life and the baby is still-born; ∝ thalassaemia minor is difficult to recognise from normal.

∝ Thalassaemia major is incompatible with life and the baby is still-born

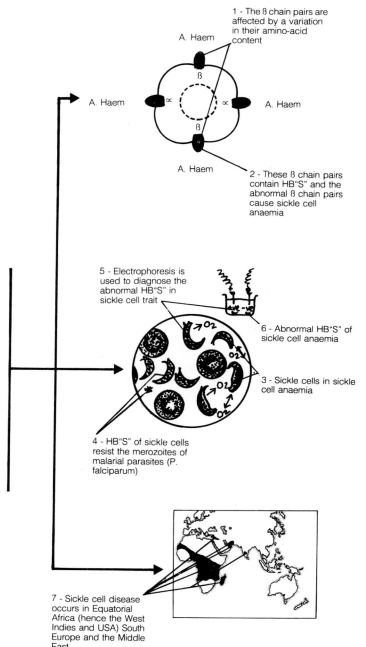

1 - The ß chain pairs are affected by a variation in their amino-acid content

A. Haem

A. Haem

A. Haem

A. Haem

ß

ß

∝

∝

2 - These ß chain pairs contain HB"S" and the abnormal ß chain pairs cause sickle cell anaemia

5 - Electrophoresis is used to diagnose the abnormal HB"S" in sickle cell trait

6 - Abnormal HB"S" of sickle cell anaemia

3 - Sickle cells in sickle cell anaemia

4 - HB"S" of sickle cells resist the merozoites of malarial parasites (P. falciparum)

7 - Sickle cell disease occurs in Equatorial Africa (hence the West Indies and USA) South Europe and the Middle East

Sickle Cell Disease – Sickle cell disease tends to occur in Equatorial Africa (thence the West Indies and USA), South Europe and the Middle East. The sickle cell gene (Hb S) mutation codes for valine (instead of glutamine) at amino acid position 6 in the ß chain of globin; this single amino acid substitution accounts for this important disease, the gene frequency of which approximates one third of the population in Equatorial Africa. Hb S may confer some resistance to parasitisation of erythrocytes by falciparum malaria; thus Hb S may have survival value.

Sickle Cell Trait – These patients are heterozygous for the Hb S gene and are usually asymptomatic, although, at low oxygen tensions, (which may include some conditions of general anaesthesia), sickling with splenic infarcts, cerebral thromboses, renal papillary necrosis and other complications may occur. Nevertheless, most of these patients have near normal life expectancies. In hospital practice, anaesthetists require to know the Hb S status of all patients from 'endemic' regions and Hb electrophoresis or a deoxygenated blood smear are performed before general anaesthesia.

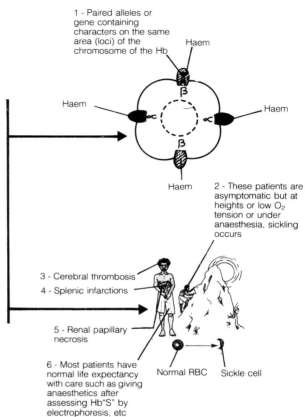

1 - Paired alleles or gene containing characters on the same area (loci) of the chromosome of the Hb

Haem

Haem

Haem

Haem

2 - These patients are asymptomatic but at heights or low O$_2$ tension or under anaesthesia, sickling occurs

3 - Cerebral thrombosis

4 - Splenic infarctions

5 - Renal papillary necrosis

6 - Most patients have normal life expectancy with care such as giving anaesthetics after assessing Hb"S" by electrophoresis, etc

Normal RBC   Sickle cell

Sickle Cell Anaemia – These are the homozygotes and these patients have no Hb A (the normal adult haemoglobin); 90% of their haemoglobin is Hb S and approximately 10% foetal Hb F.

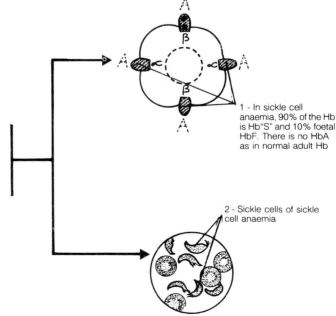

1 - In sickle cell anaemia, 90% of the Hb is Hb"S" and 10% foetal HbF. There is no HbA as in normal adult Hb

2 - Sickle cells of sickle cell anaemia

The child usually fails to thrive from approximately 6 months of age due to severe anaemia, jaundice, hepatomegaly and initially, splenomegaly. The child is often tall, thin and with a 'tower' skull. In addition to the anaemia, the patient experiences repeated episodes of vascular occlusion, (vascular occlusive crises), by masses of sickled cells with recurrent bouts of pain and fever and progressive infarction damage to the viscera, (kidney, heart, liver, bones etc).

Tropical skin ulcers, particularly on the legs, have a similar aetiology. Infections are frequent with a particular tendency to pneumococcal infections. Patients may die from infections, from aplastic crises (due to bone marrow failure) or due to widespread sickling in small blood vessels.

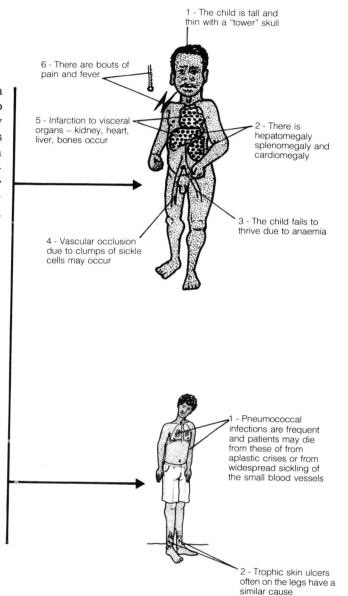

1 - The child is tall and thin with a "tower" skull

6 - There are bouts of pain and fever

5 - Infarction to visceral organs – kidney, heart, liver, bones occur

2 - There is hepatomegaly splenomegaly and cardiomegaly

3 - The child fails to thrive due to anaemia

4 - Vascular occlusion due to clumps of sickle cells may occur

1 - Pneumococcal infections are frequent and patients may die from these of from aplastic crises or from widespread sickling of the small blood vessels

2 - Trophic skin ulcers often on the legs have a similar cause

46

The blood film shows an anaemia (often normochromic, normocytic) but with anisocytosis and poikilocytosis. It is unusual to see any sickled cells on the film unless a reducing agent was added prior to the smear – this is a diagnostic test. Hb electrophoresis is diagnostic.

Any conditions which lower the pO_2 or cause an acidosis predispose to a sickling crises. No specific therapy is available but reversal of hypoxia and acidosis by alkali have a place in supportive therapy. Exchange transfusions and splenectomy are other forms of supportive therapy useful under certain conditions.

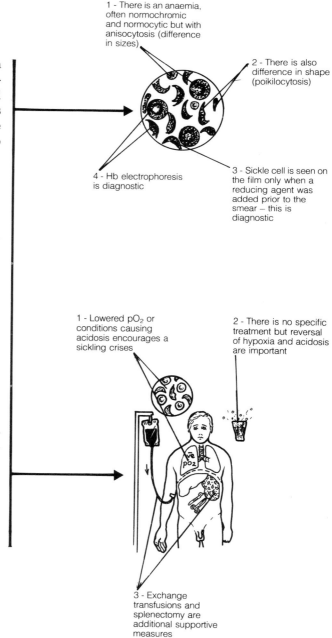

1 - There is an anaemia, often normochromic and normocytic but with anisocytosis (difference in sizes)

2 - There is also difference in shape (poikilocytosis)

3 - Sickle cell is seen on the film only when a reducing agent was added prior to the smear – this is diagnostic

4 - Hb electrophoresis is diagnostic

1 - Lowered pO_2 or conditions causing acidosis encourages a sickling crises

2 - There is no specific treatment but reversal of hypoxia and acidosis are important

3 - Exchange transfusions and splenectomy are additional supportive measures

Antibody Mediated Haemolysis – In haemolytic disease of the newborn, a Rhesus negative mother bearing Rhesus positive children is sensitised to the Rhesus antigen in her first pregnancy and during subsequent pregnancies is likely to raise high titres of antibodies capable of transplacental haemolytic disease in the foetus. Prophylactic use of anti-D at the time of first and subsequent parturitions has made a major impact on this once common and fatal disease.

In adult medicine, primary auto-immune haemolytic anaemia, a red cell auto-antibody has arisen causing haemolysis and anaemia; the Coombs' test is positive. This production of red cell

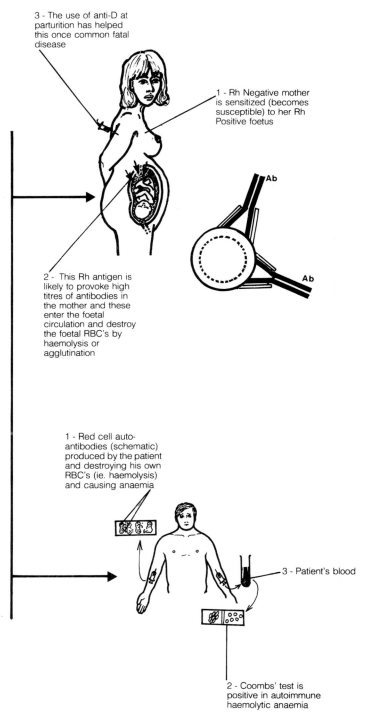

3 - The use of anti-D at parturition has helped this once common fatal disease

1 - Rh Negative mother is sensitized (becomes susceptible) to her Rh Positive foetus

Ab

Ab

2 - This Rh antigen is likely to provoke high titres of antibodies in the mother and these enter the foetal circulation and destroy the foetal RBC's by haemolysis or agglutination

1 - Red cell auto-antibodies (schematic) produced by the patient and destroying his own RBC's (ie. haemolysis) and causing anaemia

3 - Patient's blood

2 - Coombs' test is positive in autoimmune haemolytic anaemia

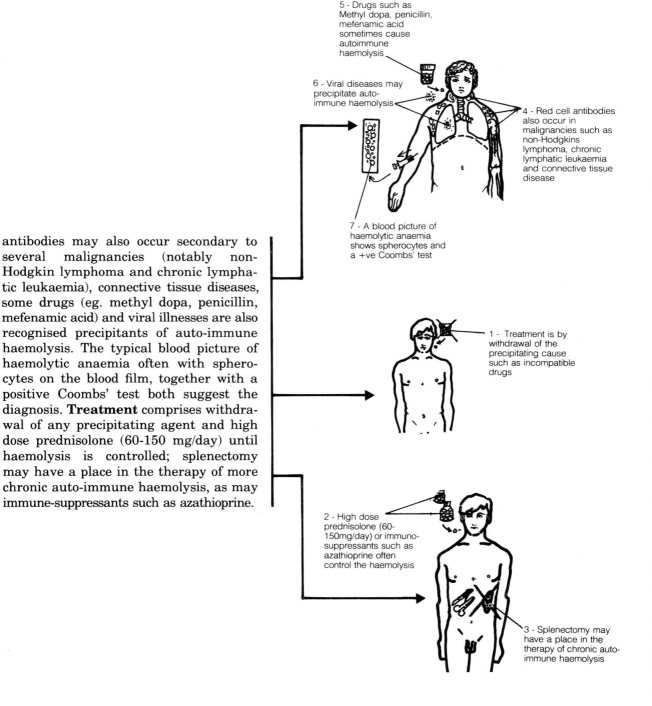

5 - Drugs such as Methyl dopa, penicillin, mefenamic acid sometimes cause autoimmune haemolysis

6 - Viral diseases may precipitate auto-immune haemolysis

4 - Red cell antibodies also occur in malignancies such as non-Hodgkins lymphoma, chronic lymphatic leukaemia and connective tissue disease

7 - A blood picture of haemolytic anaemia shows spherocytes and a +ve Coombs' test

1 - Treatment is by withdrawal of the precipitating cause such as incompatible drugs

2 - High dose prednisolone (60-150mg/day) or immuno-suppressants such as azathioprine often control the haemolysis

3 - Splenectomy may have a place in the therapy of chronic auto-immune haemolysis

antibodies may also occur secondary to several malignancies (notably non-Hodgkin lymphoma and chronic lymphatic leukaemia), connective tissue diseases, some drugs (eg. methyl dopa, penicillin, mefenamic acid) and viral illnesses are also recognised precipitants of auto-immune haemolysis. The typical blood picture of haemolytic anaemia often with spherocytes on the blood film, together with a positive Coombs' test both suggest the diagnosis. **Treatment** comprises withdrawal of any precipitating agent and high dose prednisolone (60-150 mg/day) until haemolysis is controlled; splenectomy may have a place in the therapy of more chronic auto-immune haemolysis, as may immune-suppressants such as azathioprine.

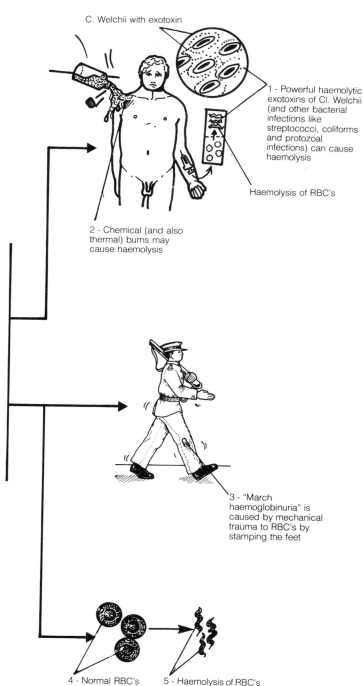

C. Welchii with exotoxin

1 - Powerful haemolytic exotoxins of Cl. Welchii (and other bacterial infections like streptococci, coliforms and protozoal infections) can cause haemolysis

Haemolysis of RBC's

2 - Chemical (and also thermal) burns may cause haemolysis

3 - "March haemoglobinuria" is caused by mechanical trauma to RBC's by stamping the feet

4 - Normal RBC's   5 - Haemolysis of RBC's

Extra-corpuscular Causes of Haemolysis (not mediated by antibody) – The powerful haemolytic exotoxin of *Cl. Welchii* accounts for the potentially severe haemolysis that may occur in this clostridial infection; other bacterial infections may also be accompanied by haemolysis (eg. streptococci, coliforms) as may protozoal infections (eg. malarial 'blackwater fever'). Thermal burns and chemicals (eg. benzene derivatives) may cause haemolysis – perhaps severe intravascular haemolysis, and the curious condition of march haemoglobinuria is caused by mechanical trauma to red cells by stamping of the feet!

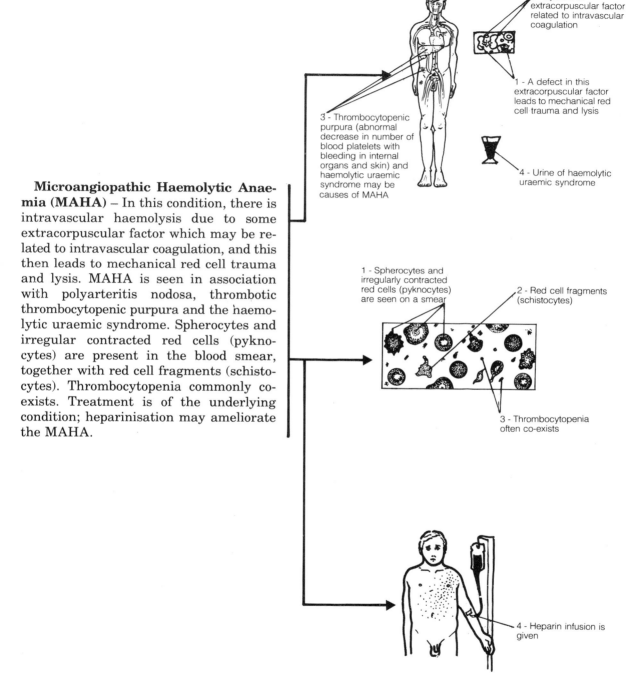

2 - Symbol of extracorpuscular factor related to intravascular coagulation

1 - A defect in this extracorpuscular factor leads to mechanical red cell trauma and lysis

3 - Thrombocytopenic purpura (abnormal decrease in number of blood platelets with bleeding in internal organs and skin) and haemolytic uraemic syndrome may be causes of MAHA

4 - Urine of haemolytic uraemic syndrome

1 - Spherocytes and irregularly contracted red cells (pyknocytes) are seen on a smear

2 - Red cell fragments (schistocytes)

3 - Thrombocytopenia often co-exists

4 - Heparin infusion is given

Microangiopathic Haemolytic Anaemia (MAHA) – In this condition, there is intravascular haemolysis due to some extracorpuscular factor which may be related to intravascular coagulation, and this then leads to mechanical red cell trauma and lysis. MAHA is seen in association with polyarteritis nodosa, thrombotic thrombocytopenic purpura and the haemolytic uraemic syndrome. Spherocytes and irregular contracted red cells (pyknocytes) are present in the blood smear, together with red cell fragments (schistocytes). Thrombocytopenia commonly co-exists. Treatment is of the underlying condition; heparinisation may ameliorate the MAHA.

HAEMORRHAGIC DISEASES

Following the infliction of a superficial cut, vasoconstriction of the surrounding arterioles lessens the bleeding before a platelet 'plug' forms. At first this platelet plug is only loosely held together and is unstable. It is secondary haemostasis brought about by the coagulation cascade, which effects permanent haemostasis.

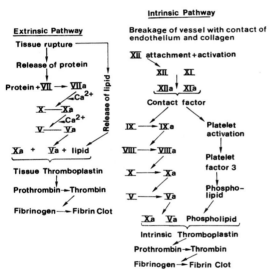

Extrinsic Pathway

Tissue rupture

Release of protein

Protein + $\underline{VII}$ ⟶ $\underline{VIIa}$

Release of lipid

$\underline{X}$ ⟶ $\underline{Xa}$ — Ca^{2+}

$\underline{V}$ ⟶ $\underline{Va}$ — Ca^{2+}

$\underline{Xa}$ + $\underline{Va}$ + lipid

Tissue Thromboplastin

Prothrombin ⟶ Thrombin

Fibrinogen ⟶ Fibrin Clot

Intrinsic Pathway

Breakage of vessel with contact of endothelium and collagen

$\underline{XII}$ attachment + activation

$\underline{XII}$ $\underline{XI}$

$\underline{XIIa}$ $\underline{XIa}$

Contact factor

$\underline{IX}$ ⟶ $\underline{IXa}$ Platelet activation

$\underline{VIII}$ ⟶ $\underline{VIIIa}$

$\underline{X}$ ⟶ $\underline{Xa}$ Platelet factor 3

$\underline{V}$ ⟶ $\underline{Va}$ Phospholipid

$\underline{Xa}$ $\underline{Va}$ Phospholipid

Intrinsic Thromboplastin

Prothrombin ⟶ Thrombin

Fibrinogen ⟶ Fibrin Clot

The coagulation cascade is an amplification system where an initial trigger to coagulation activates a coagulation factor, (each numbered with a Roman numeral) which activates another factor and so forth, prothrombin being activated to thrombin which splits fibrinogen to form the fibrin clot. The system is amplified at each step so that a powerful coagulation activity is generated. It will be noted that both calcium and phospholipid are required for coagulation.

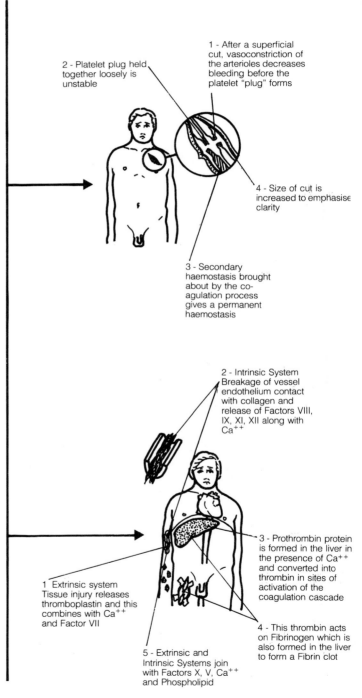

2 - Platelet plug held together loosely is unstable

1 - After a superficial cut, vasoconstriction of the arterioles decreases bleeding before the platelet "plug" forms

4 - Size of cut is increased to emphasise clarity

3 - Secondary haemostasis brought about by the co-agulation process gives a permanent haemostasis

2 - Intrinsic System Breakage of vessel endothelium contact with collagen and release of Factors VIII, IX, XI, XII along with Ca^{++}

1 Extrinsic system Tissue injury releases thromboplastin and this combines with Ca^{++} and Factor VII

3 - Prothrombin protein is formed in the liver in the presence of Ca^{++} and converted into thrombin in sites of activation of the coagulation cascade

4 - This thrombin acts on Fibrinogen which is also formed in the liver to form a Fibrin clot

5 - Extrinsic and Intrinsic Systems join with Factors X, V, Ca^{++} and Phospholipid

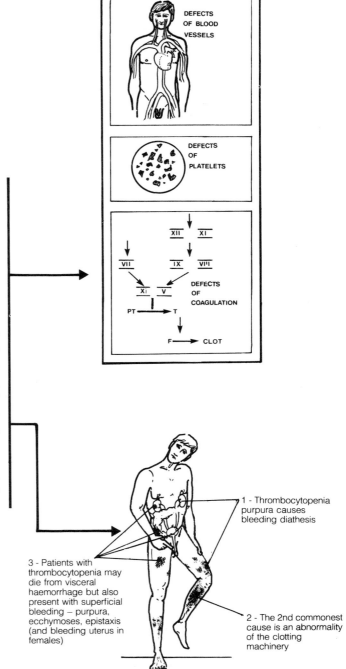

It will be clear from the above description that haemorrhagic diseases could arise from defects in the blood vessels, the platelets and/or the coagulation (clotting) factors. The **commonest cause** of bleeding diathesis is due to thrombocytopenia and the second commonest cause is an abnormality of the clotting machinery. Bleeding due to thrombocytopenia tends to begin after a very short or absent latency, (because of the platelet plug's primary role). Patients with thrombocytopenia may die from visceral haemorrhage but tend to present with spontaneous superficial bleeding – purpura, ecchymoses, bleeding from epithelium (eg. nose, uterus). Patients with coagulation defects usually present with bleeding, usually following trauma, into deep tissues – muscles, joints, viscera, and often after a longer latent period, (because the coagulation cascade is concerned with secondary haemostasis).

MAJOR CAUSES OF BLEEDING DISORDERS

DEFECTS OF BLOOD VESSELS

DEFECTS OF PLATELETS

DEFECTS OF COAGULATION

1 - Thrombocytopenia purpura causes bleeding diathesis

2 - The 2nd commonest cause is an abnormality of the clotting machinery

3 - Patients with thrombocytopenia may die from visceral haemorrhage but also present with superficial bleeding – purpura, ecchymoses, epistaxis (and bleeding uterus in females)

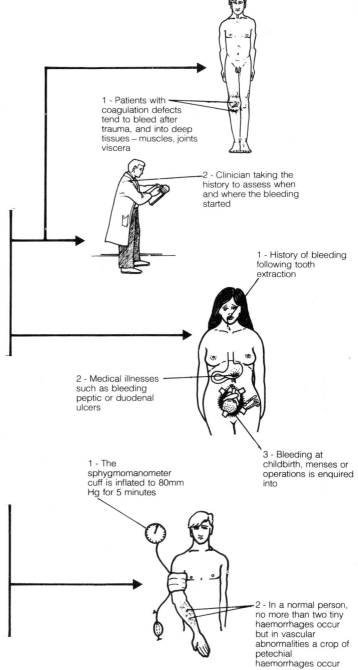

1 - Patients with coagulation defects tend to bleed after trauma, and into deep tissues – muscles, joints viscera

2 - Clinician taking the history to assess when and where the bleeding started

1 - History of bleeding following tooth extraction

2 - Medical illnesses such as bleeding peptic or duodenal ulcers

3 - Bleeding at childbirth, menses or operations is enquired into

1 - The sphygmomanometer cuff is inflated to 80mm Hg for 5 minutes

2 - In a normal person, no more than two tiny haemorrhages occur but in vascular abnormalities a crop of petechial haemorrhages occur

The **clinical history** may give insight into the type of bleeding diathesis. The clinician always enquires as when the bleeding started and from where it commenced.

He specifically enquires as to whether there has been a history of bleeding tendency in the past – eg. following tooth extraction, childbirth, menses or operations and he enquires for other medical illness and medications being taken.

The **investigation** of bleeding diathesis begins with a **Hess test**. This is a test of small blood vessel fragility. A sphygmomanometer cuff is applied to the upper arm and inflated to 80mm Hg for five minutes. In a normal person, no more than two tiny skin haemorrhages will occur; in vascular abnormalities a crop of petechiae occur. The second clinical investigation that may be useful is the bleeding time – an approximate indicator of primary haemostasis; (it is not prolonged by coagulation disorders). Here, a sphygmomanometer cuff is inflated to 40mm Hg and a stiletto needle is used to make three transdermal punctures on the volar aspect of the forearm. A piece of filter paper is used to blot the puncture sites every 30 seconds until haemostasis ceases and the average time recorded; the normal bleeding time is less than seven minutes.

1 - Here the sphygmomanometer cuff is inflated to 40mm Hg

3 - A filter paper blots the site of puncture every 30 seconds until haemostasis occurs and the average time recorded – it is about 7 minutes

2 - A stiletto needle is used to make 3 transdermal punctures on the volar (palmar) aspect of forearm

Another approximate but useful bedside investigation is the whole blood clotting time: venous blood is decanted into 3 glass tubes and inverted every fifteen seconds at 37°C until clotting occurs; the average time is recorded and should be less than seven minutes; this is a crude test of the intrinsic clotting pathway.

2 - Test tubes are inverted every 15 seconds at 37°C

1 - Venous blood is decanted into 3 glass tubes and inverted every 15 seconds at 37°C until clotting occurs

3 - Finally clotting occurs and should be less than 7 minutes – a crude test of intrinsic clotting time

The laboratory tests are more decisive and diagnostic, but the student must be aware of the bedside methods just described. An estimate of the platelet count by a blood film or an automated count is the

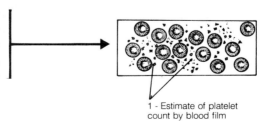

1 - Estimate of platelet count by blood film

first essential investigation, to be followed by an assessment of megakaryocyte numbers in the sternal marrow aspirate if there is thrombocytopenia. More complex platelet function tests exist if the abnormality appears to be with the platelets and their numbers are normal.

The delineation of an abnormality in the coagulation cascade depends upon several laboratory tests; (in the following description, normal values are not given as simultaneous laboratory control samples give these on each occasion). The prothrombin time (**PT**) tests the whole extrinsic system: in this test, tissue thromboplastin is added to plasma, the plasma is re-calcified and the clotting time noted. The P.T. is prolonged by deficiency of one or more of the following factors: VII, X, V, prothrombin and (to a lesser degree) fibrinogen, and also in the presence of heparin and fibrin degradation products (**FDP**).

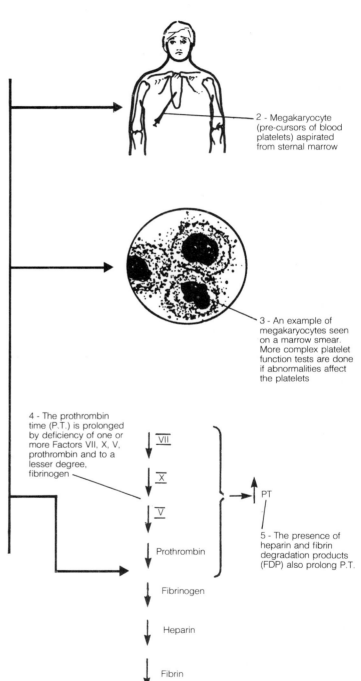

2 - Megakaryocyte (pre-cursors of blood platelets) aspirated from sternal marrow

3 - An example of megakaryocytes seen on a marrow smear. More complex platelet function tests are done if abnormalities affect the platelets

4 - The prothrombin time (P.T.) is prolonged by deficiency of one or more Factors VII, X, V, prothrombin and to a lesser degree, fibrinogen

VII

X

V

Prothrombin

Fibrinogen

Heparin

Fibrin

PT

5 - The presence of heparin and fibrin degradation products (FDP) also prolong P.T.

In the partial thromboplastin time with kaolin (**KPTT**) or kaolin cephalin clotting time (**KCCT**), phospholipid and kaolin are used to activate or by-pass factor XII and the time of clotting of the blood sample reflects the integrity of the intrinsic coagulation pathway. The KPTT is prolonged in deficiencies of IX, VII, X, V, prothrombin and fibrinogen, and also in the presence of heparin and FDP.

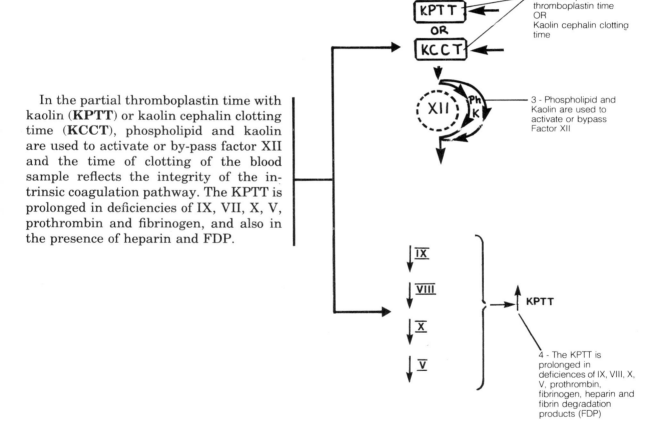

1 - Factor XII being by-passed

2 - Kaolin partial thromboplastin time
OR
Kaolin cephalin clotting time

3 - Phospholipid and Kaolin are used to activate or bypass Factor XII

4 - The KPTT is prolonged in deficiences of IX, VIII, X, V, prothrombin, fibrinogen, heparin and fibrin degradation products (FDP)

The thrombin time (**TT**) tests the conversion of fibrinogen to fibrin. It is prolonged by deficiency or abnormality of fibrinogen and by heparin and FDP. The measurement of fibrinogen titre is useful as it is typically low in disseminated **intravascular coagulopathy (DIC)**. Also in DIC, there are high circulating levels of fibrin degradation products (FDP) and their measurement is also diagnostically important.

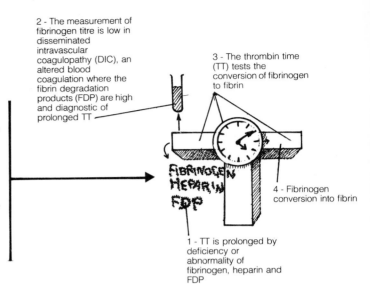

2 - The measurement of fibrinogen titre is low in disseminated intravascular coagulopathy (DIC), an altered blood coagulation where the fibrin degradation products (FDP) are high and diagnostic of prolonged TT

3 - The thrombin time (TT) tests the conversion of fibrinogen to fibrin

4 - Fibrinogen conversion into fibrin

1 - TT is prolonged by deficiency or abnormality of fibrinogen, heparin and FDP

Disorders of Primary Haemostasis – Some vascular disorders are common but fortunately lead to only minor bleeding diatheses. Examples are the purpura seen in old age and in Cushing's syndrome, both due to vascular fragility. Hereditary telangiectasia and Ehlers-Danlos syndrome are rare examples. Scurvy and anaphylactoid purpura would come within this group.

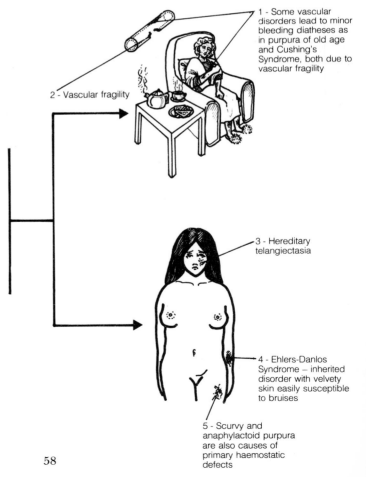

1 - Some vascular disorders lead to minor bleeding diatheses as in purpura of old age and Cushing's Syndrome, both due to vascular fragility

2 - Vascular fragility

3 - Hereditary telangiectasia

4 - Ehlers-Danlos Syndrome – inherited disorder with velvety skin easily susceptible to bruises

5 - Scurvy and anaphylactoid purpura are also causes of primary haemostatic defects

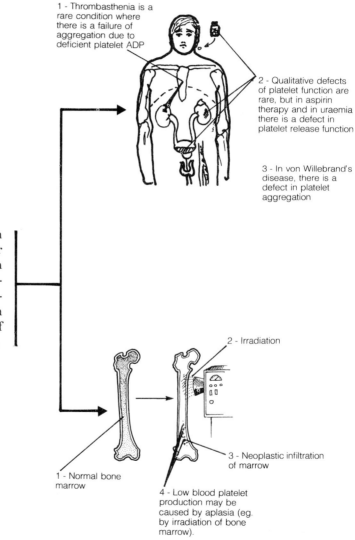

1 - Thrombasthenia is a rare condition where there is a failure of aggregation due to deficient platelet ADP

2 - Qualitative defects of platelet function are rare, but in aspirin therapy and in uraemia there is a defect in platelet release function

3 - In von Willebrand's disease, there is a defect in platelet aggregation

Qualitative defects of platelet function are uncommon, although in uraemia or during aspirin therapy there is a defect in platelet release function. In von Willebrand's disease there is a defect in platelet aggregation. In the rare condition thrombasthenia, there is a failure of aggregation due to deficient platelet ADP.

2 - Irradiation

3 - Neoplastic infiltration of marrow

1 - Normal bone marrow

4 - Low blood platelet production may be caused by aplasia (eg. by irradiation of bone marrow).

Much more common are the causes of low platelet numbers (thrombocytopenia). The causes may be failure of production (aplastic, suppressed or infiltrated marrow) or excessive destruction. In **idiopathic thrombocytopenic purpura (ITP),** platelet auto-antibodies occur, (for no known reason) and destroy peripheral blood platelets leading to a bleeding diathesis; the marrow contains many active megakaryocytes. Treatment is with high dose steroids (prednisolone).

Auto-antibodies to platelets also occur in several other diseases (eg. SLE, chronic lymphatic leukaemia, auto-immune haemolytic anaemia) and in a few patients on certain drugs (eg. sedormid). Platelets are also consumed in large, active spleens (hypersplenism) and by large haemangiomas.

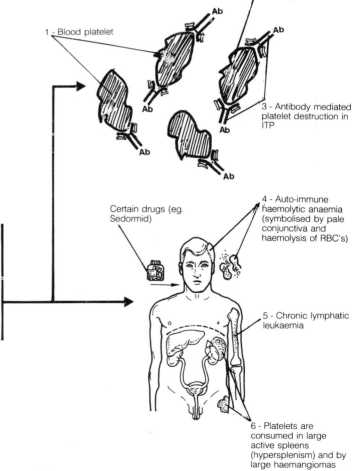

4 - Treatment is by high dose of steroids eg. Prednisolone 20-30mg daily

2 - In ITP platelet auto-antibodies occur and destroy the peripheral blood platelets leading to a bleeding diathesis like purpura

1 - Idiopathic thrombocytopenic purpura

3 - The marrow contains many active megakaryocytes

1 - Blood platelet

2 - Blood platelet

3 - Antibody mediated platelet destruction in ITP

Certain drugs (eg. Sedormid)

4 - Auto-immune haemolytic anaemia (symbolised by pale conjunctiva and haemolysis of RBC's)

5 - Chronic lymphatic leukaemia

6 - Platelets are consumed in large active spleens (hypersplenism) and by large haemangiomas

The disorders of coagulation may be divided into congenital disorders (of which the most important two, haemophilia and Christmas disease, will be discussed) and acquired disorders, (notably vitamin K deficiency, disseminated intravascular coagulation, liver disease, anti-coagulant drugs etc.).

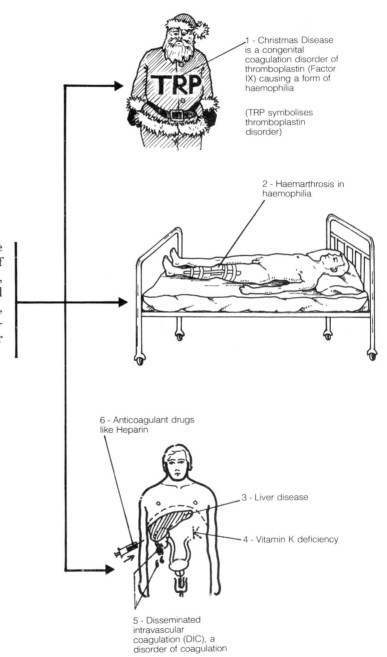

1 - Christmas Disease is a congenital coagulation disorder of thromboplastin (Factor IX) causing a form of haemophilia

(TRP symbolises thromboplastin disorder)

2 - Haemarthrosis in haemophilia

6 - Anticoagulant drugs like Heparin

3 - Liver disease

4 - Vitamin K deficiency

5 - Disseminated intravascular coagulation (DIC), a disorder of coagulation

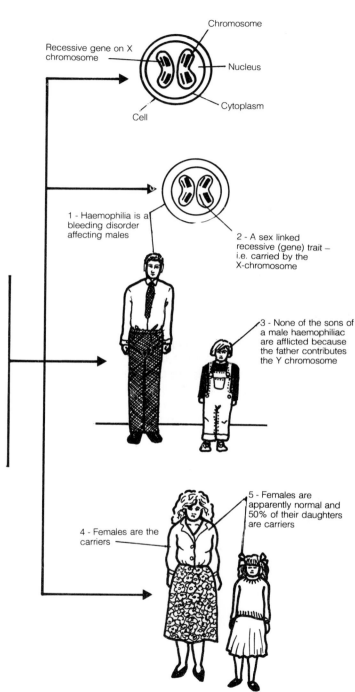

Recessive gene on X chromosome

Chromosome

Nucleus

Cytoplasm

Cell

1 - Haemophilia is a bleeding disorder affecting males

2 - A sex linked recessive (gene) trait — i.e. carried by the X-chromosome

3 - None of the sons of a male haemophiliac are afflicted because the father contributes the Y chromosome

4 - Females are the carriers

5 - Females are apparently normal and 50% of their daughters are carriers

Haemophilia

Haemophilia is a bleeding disorder that affects males and is transmitted by apparently normal females (ie. a sex linked **recessive trait affecting none of the sons of a male haemophiliac; all his daughters are carriers**). Affected males are deficient in factor VIII activity although the severity of this deficiency varies considerably accounting for the varying severity of clinical haemophilia. Although patients may be present at birth, they usually present later with easy bruising as the child learns to crawl. With the eruption of the primary dentition, injuries to the tongue and lips may result in prolonged haemorrhage. Haemarthroses, (especially of knees, elbows and ankles), the hallmark of severe haemophilia, start occurring when the child starts to walk and by the time the child is ten years old he will usually have experienced several episodes of prolonged bleeding from wounds, haemarthroses, intramuscular haematomas, haematuria, epistaxes and gastrointestinal bleeding. Any surgical procedure (eg. circumcision, tonsillectomy) may lead to dangerous haemorrhage and the child is prone to visceral bleeding after trauma.

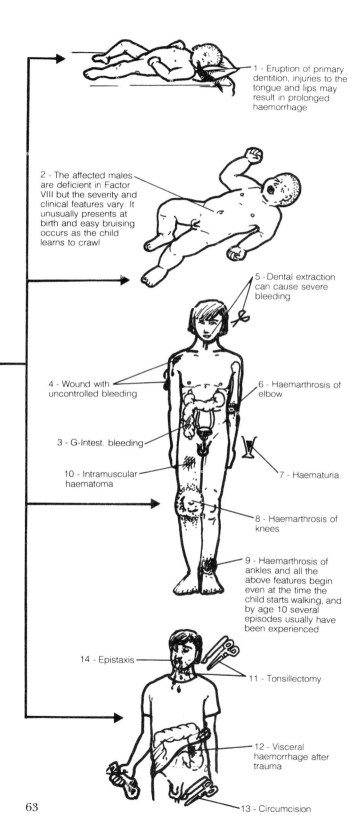

1 - Eruption of primary dentition, injuries to the tongue and lips may result in prolonged haemorrhage

2 - The affected males are deficient in Factor VIII but the severity and clinical features vary. It unusually presents at birth and easy bruising occurs as the child learns to crawl

5 - Dental extraction can cause severe bleeding

4 - Wound with uncontrolled bleeding

6 - Haemarthrosis of elbow

3 - G-Intest. bleeding

7 - Haematuria

10 - Intramuscular haematoma

8 - Haemarthrosis of knees

9 - Haemarthrosis of ankles and all the above features begin even at the time the child starts walking, and by age 10 several episodes usually have been experienced

14 - Epistaxis

11 - Tonsillectomy

12 - Visceral haemorrhage after trauma

13 - Circumcision

Although fresh blood and fresh frozen plasma both contain factor VIII activity, it is only since the widespread availability of factor VIII concentrate (cryoprecipitate) that a powerful treatment for haemophilia has become available. For a haemarthrosis, the joint is splinted and lightly bandaged and protected while cryoprecipitate is given intravenously to raise the factor VIII level to at least 40% of normal; aspiration of the joint may be necessary later. Similarly, cryoprecipitate infusion would precede any elective surgery.

Transfer Pack FKGP
E 0516

2 - Factor VIII concentrate (cryoprecipitate) is a powerful treatment for haemophilia and is given I.V.

3 - The cryoprecipitate given I.V. should raise Factor VIII to at least 40% of normal.

1 - In haemarthrosis, the joint is splinted and lightly bandaged to protect it

4 - Aspiration of the joint may be necessary later

Christmas disease is also a sex-linked recessive condition but much less common than haemophilia. Factor IX is deficient in Christmas disease and as factor IX is more stable than factor VIII, fresh frozen plasma or factor IX concentrate may be used to elevate the factor IX level.

In addition to the abnormality of primary haemostasis already described in von Willebrand's disease, there is a low factor VIII activity and cryoprecipitate may also be required here.

1 - Christmas disease is also a sex-linked recessive condition due to Factor IX deficiency (Schematic!)

2 - Bleeding is controlled by infusion of fresh frozen plasma or Factor IX concentrate to elevate Factor IX level

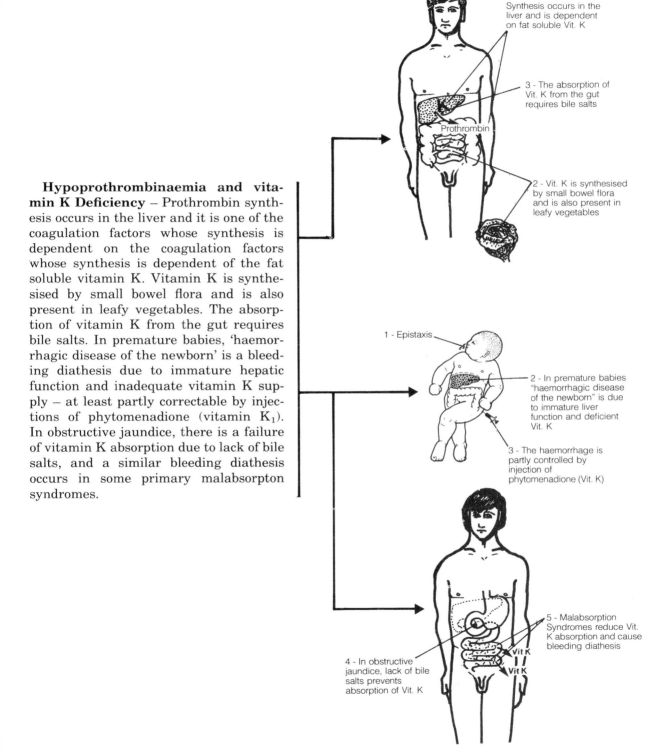

1 - Prothrombin
Synthesis occurs in the
liver and is dependent
on fat soluble Vit. K

3 - The absorption of
Vit. K from the gut
requires bile salts

Prothrombin

2 - Vit. K is synthesised
by small bowel flora
and is also present in
leafy vegetables

1 - Epistaxis

2 - In premature babies
"haemorrhagic disease
of the newborn" is due
to immature liver
function and deficient
Vit. K

3 - The haemorrhage is
partly controlled by
injection of
phytomenadione (Vit. K)

5 - Malabsorption
Syndromes reduce Vit.
K absorption and cause
bleeding diathesis

Vit K
Vit K

4 - In obstructive
jaundice, lack of bile
salts prevents
absorption of Vit. K

Hypoprothrombinaemia and vitamin K Deficiency – Prothrombin synthesis occurs in the liver and it is one of the coagulation factors whose synthesis is dependent on the coagulation factors whose synthesis is dependent of the fat soluble vitamin K. Vitamin K is synthesised by small bowel flora and is also present in leafy vegetables. The absorption of vitamin K from the gut requires bile salts. In premature babies, 'haemorrhagic disease of the newborn' is a bleeding diathesis due to immature hepatic function and inadequate vitamin K supply – at least partly correctable by injections of phytomenadione (vitamin K_1). In obstructive jaundice, there is a failure of vitamin K absorption due to lack of bile salts, and a similar bleeding diathesis occurs in some primary malabsorpton syndromes.

In severe hepatic disease, the synthesis of vitamin K dependent coagulation factors (including prothrombin) is deficient and a coagulation defect results.

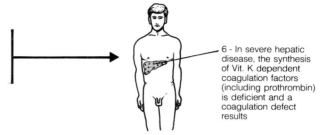

6 - In severe hepatic disease, the synthesis of Vit. K dependent coagulation factors (including prothrombin) is deficient and a coagulation defect results

ANTICOAGULANTS

Anticoagulant drugs are used in the prophylaxis and treatment of thrombo-embolic conditions. In general, anticoagulants should be avoided in patients with peptic ulcer, uncontrolled hypertension and in the elderly – all of whom have an increased tendency to bleed. These drugs should also be avoided in the first few days after surgery.

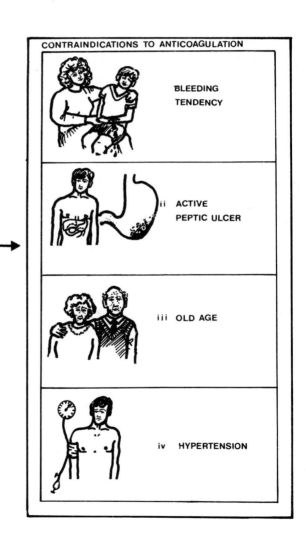

CONTRAINDICATIONS TO ANTICOAGULATION

BLEEDING TENDENCY

ii ACTIVE PEPTIC ULCER

iii OLD AGE

iv HYPERTENSION

Heparin – Heparin is a sulphur-containing mucopolysaccharide that is a potent inhibitor at several sites in the coagulation cascade. It is administered by subcutaneous injection (for low dose prophylaxis against DVT eg. 5000 units bd-tds) or by continuous infusion in 0.9% saline (for high dose therapy eg. 40,000 units daily); its anticoagulant effects are immediate. Although the whole blood clotting time is a crude indicator of anticoagulation by heparin, the thrombin time test is the preferred monitor of heparin therapy. Protamine sulphate is an antidote for heparin and with a reasonable therapeutic dose of heparin, the prolongation of the **in vitro** thrombin time is correctable to normal by 2 mg/ml protamine but not by 1mg/ml. Apart from haemorrhage, heparin can produce a pyrexia and occasionally a hypersensitivity reaction. Transient alopecia and thrombocytopenia have also been reported.

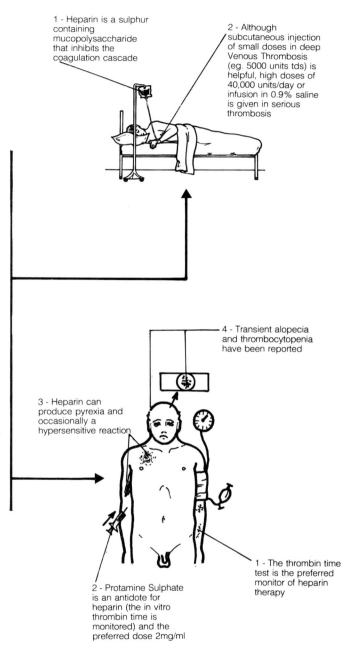

1 - Heparin is a sulphur containing mucopolysaccharide that inhibits the coagulation cascade

2 - Although subcutaneous injection of small doses in deep Venous Thrombosis (eg. 5000 units tds) is helpful, high doses of 40,000 units/day or infusion in 0.9% saline is given in serious thrombosis

4 - Transient alopecia and thrombocytopenia have been reported

3 - Heparin can produce pyrexia and occasionally a hypersensitive reaction

1 - The thrombin time test is the preferred monitor of heparin therapy

2 - Protamine Sulphate is an antidote for heparin (the in vitro thrombin time is monitored) and the preferred dose 2mg/ml

Coumarins – These agents are orally active and block the action of vitamin K and the synthesis of prothrombin. Their action is delayed until the circulating levels of these factors fall due to biological decay, and although the half-life of factor VII may be as short as five hours and the prothrombin time (PT) be prolonged early after coumarin administration, nevertheless, the anti-thrombotic effectiveness may not occur for 48 hours, when factor X levels have fallen. Warfarin is the most popular coumarin and seems to have no side effects other than haemorrhage. Warfarin anticoagulation is commenced in adults with an initial dose of 12-15 mg with 10 mg orally on the second and third days. Thereafter, the maintenance dose, (usually 2.5-7.5 mg daily) is monitored by frequent P.T. estimations; the ideal prolongation recommended depends to some degree on the laboratory methodology – say 2-4 × normal). The anticoagulant effects of warfarin may be immediately reversed by an infusion of fresh frozen plasma and more slowly antagonised by vitamin K injections.

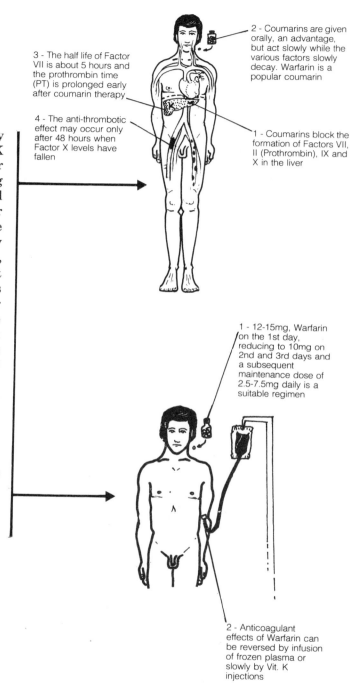

2 - Coumarins are given orally, an advantage, but act slowly while the various factors slowly decay. Warfarin is a popular coumarin

3 - The half life of Factor VII is about 5 hours and the prothrombin time (PT) is prolonged early after coumarin therapy

4 - The anti-thrombotic effect may occur only after 48 hours when Factor X levels have fallen

1 - Coumarins block the formation of Factors VII, II (Prothrombin), IX and X in the liver

1 - 12-15mg, Warfarin on the 1st day, reducing to 10mg on 2nd and 3rd days and a subsequent maintenance dose of 2.5-7.5mg daily is a suitable regimen

2 - Anticoagulant effects of Warfarin can be reversed by infusion of frozen plasma or slowly by Vit. K injections

Various drugs may interfere with anti-coagulant stabilisation. Thus antibiotic administration to patients with a marginal vitamin K intake may render these patients vitamin K deficient and warfarin sensitive. Phenylbutazone displaces warfarin from plasma protein binding sites and inhibits its liver microsomal metabolism, both tending to increase warfarin activity, whereas enzyme-inducing drugs (eg. barbiturates) may decrease warfarin activity by induction of its faster catabolism.

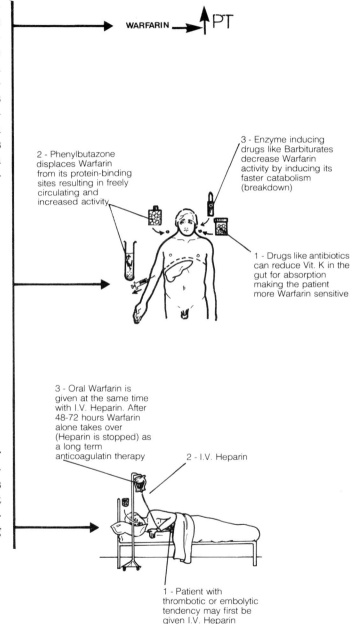

WARFARIN → ↑ PT

2 - Phenylbutazone displaces Warfarin from its protein-binding sites resulting in freely circulating and increased activity

3 - Enzyme inducing drugs like Barbiturates decrease Warfarin activity by inducing its faster catabolism (breakdown)

1 - Drugs like antibiotics can reduce Vit. K in the gut for absorption making the patient more Warfarin sensitive

3 - Oral Warfarin is given at the same time with I.V. Heparin. After 48-72 hours Warfarin alone takes over (Heparin is stopped) as a long term anticoagulatin therapy

2 - I.V. Heparin

1 - Patient with thrombotic or embolytic tendency may first be given I.V. Heparin

In patients with a serious thrombotic or embolic tendency, it is customary to initiate anticoagulation with intravenous heparin, whilst starting oral warfarin at the same time. By 48-72 hours, the warfarin takes over as the method of long term maintenance anticoagulation.

Disseminated Intravascular Coagulopathy (DIC) – This condition with widespread clotting within the vascular network may be caused by materials with tissue thromboplastic properties. This seems to be the mechanism in several complicated obstetric conditions (eg. amniotic fluid embolism, premature placental separation, and retained dead foetus), in association with massive tissue trauma and in certain malignancies well-recognised to be associated with DIC, (eg. acute promyelocytic leukaemia, disseminated mucus secreting adenocarcinoma – especially of pancreatic or GI tract origin). In septicaemia due to Gram negative bacilli, DIC may be due to endotoxin damage to platelets and vascular endothelium, and factor VII activation. Antigen-antibody reactions (immune complexing) may also trigger DIC.

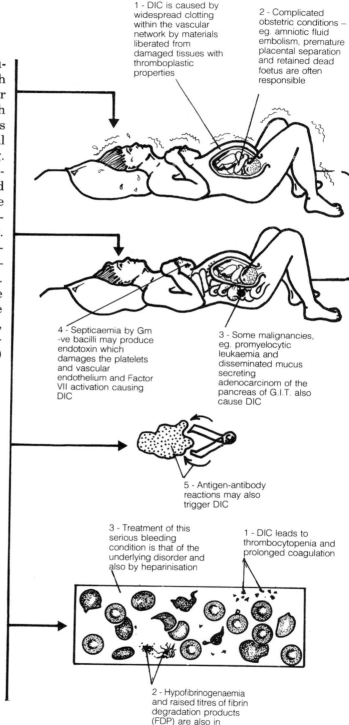

1 - DIC is caused by widespread clotting within the vascular network by materials liberated from damaged tissues with thromboplastic properties

2 - Complicated obstetric conditions – eg. amniotic fluid embolism, premature placental separation and retained dead foetus are often responsible

4 - Septicaemia by Gm -ve bacilli may produce endotoxin which damages the platelets and vascular endothelium and Factor VII activation causing DIC

3 - Some malignancies, eg. promyelocytic leukaemia and disseminated mucus secreting adenocarcinom of the pancreas of G.I.T. also cause DIC

5 - Antigen-antibody reactions may also trigger DIC

3 - Treatment of this serious bleeding condition is that of the underlying disorder and also by heparinisation

1 - DIC leads to thrombocytopenia and prolonged coagulation

2 - Hypofibrinogenaemia and raised titres of fibrin degradation products (FDP) are also in evidence

The massive intravascular clotting leads to thrombocytopenia, prolonged coagulation tests, hypofibrinogenaemia and raised titres of fibrin degradation products (FDP). The treatment of this dangerous condition associated with serious bleeding (due to the secondary deficiency in haemostatic mechanisms) is the treatment of the underlying disorder and perhaps, careful heparinisation.

THE LEUKAEMIAS

The term leukaemia is used to describe bone marrow malignancy involving cells of the leucocyte family which spill over into the peripheral blood. Although in lower mammals a viral aetiology is probable, this is not proven in humans, and although there is a proven increased incidence of leukaemias following radiation (and cytotoxic chemical mutagens), this does not fully explain the aetiology of human leukaemia. There is an increased incidence of leukaemia in Down's syndrome (trisomy 21) and certain other rare congenital syndromes (eg. Fanconi's anaemia, Bloom's syndrome).

Leukaemia is classified by the series of white cells involved and by the rapidity of growth (acute versus chronic).

Acute Lymphoblastic Leukaemia (ALL) – This is a disease that most commonly afflicts children, who present to medical attention with symptoms referable to bone marrow failure. The diagnosis should be suspected in any child who presents with anaemia, bruising or lymphadenopathy. The blood count may

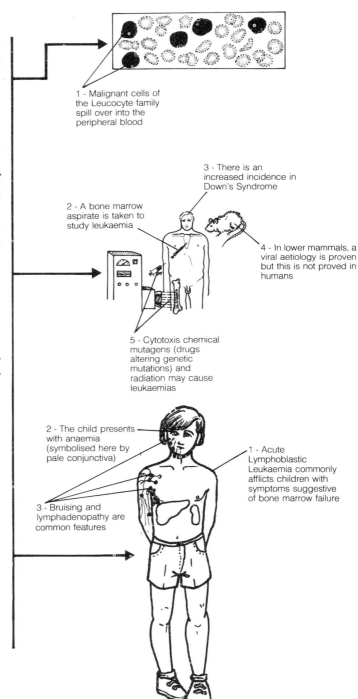

1 - Malignant cells of the Leucocyte family spill over into the peripheral blood

3 - There is an increased incidence in Down's Syndrome

2 - A bone marrow aspirate is taken to study leukaemia

4 - In lower mammals, a viral aetiology is proven but this is not proved in humans

5 - Cytotoxis chemical mutagens (drugs altering genetic mutations) and radiation may cause leukaemias

2 - The child presents with anaemia (symbolised here by pale conjunctiva)

1 - Acute Lymphoblastic Leukaemia commonly afflicts children with symptoms suggestive of bone marrow failure

3 - Bruising and lymphadenopathy are common features

show anaemia and thrombocytopenia and the white cell count may be normal or raised. However, the neutrophil count is frequently low and lymphoblasts may be seen on the blood film. The diagnosis is confirmed by examination of the bone marrow which shows excessive numbers of lymphoblasts.

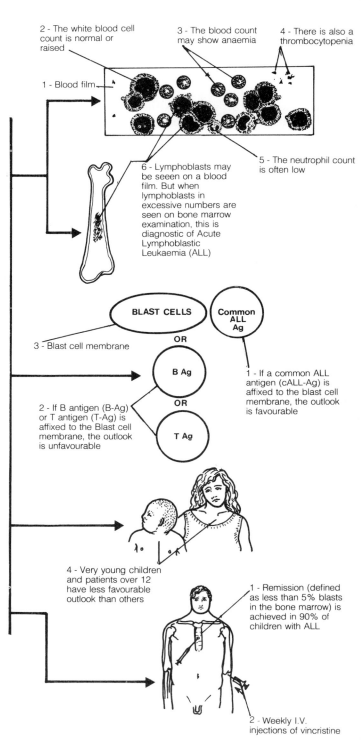

2 - The white blood cell count is normal or raised

3 - The blood count may show anaemia

4 - There is also a thrombocytopenia

1 - Blood film

5 - The neutrophil count is often low

6 - Lymphoblasts may be seeen on a blood film. But when lymphoblasts in excessive numbers are seen on bone marrow examination, this is diagnostic of Acute Lymphoblastic Leukaemia (ALL)

BLAST CELLS

Common ALL Ag

3 - Blast cell membrane

B Ag

OR

T Ag

OR

1 - If a common ALL antigen (cALL-Ag) is affixed to the blast cell membrane, the outlook is favourable

2 - If B antigen (B-Ag) or T antigen (T-Ag) is affixed to the Blast cell membrane, the outlook is unfavourable

ALL can be subcategorised by lymphoblast morphology and cytochemistry but the most important prognostic indicators are the possession by the cells of common ALL antigen, cALLA, (favourable outlook), or B or T cell antigenic determinants (unfavourable outlook), on their cell membranes. Very young children and patients beyond the age of 12 years have a slightly less favourable outlook than others/blast count at presentation also fare worse.

4 - Very young children and patients over 12 have less favourable outlook than others

1 - Remission (defined as less than 5% blasts in the bone marrow) is achieved in 90% of children with ALL

2 - Weekly I.V. injections of vincristine

It is now possible to achieve remission, (confirmed by a bone marrow showing less than 5% lymphoblasts), within 4-6 weeks in 90% of children with ALL (and the majority of adults too), using a combination of oral prednisolone, weekly intravenous vincristine and usually a third drug, (daunorubicin or asparaginase – or both in some 'intensive' induction schemes). During the initiation of treatment, there may be a massive breakdown of leukaemia cells with hyperkalaemia and hyperuricaemia with the possibilities of cardiac dysrhythmias and urate nephropathy. These complications can usually be avoided by adequate hydration of the patient, administration of allopurinol, (an inhibitor of xanthine oxidase and hence urate formation), and sometimes alkalinisation of the urine.

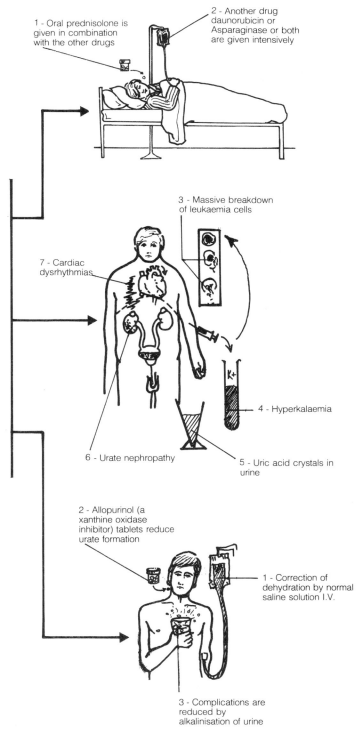

1 - Oral prednisolone is given in combination with the other drugs

2 - Another drug daunorubicin or Asparaginase or both are given intensively

3 - Massive breakdown of leukaemia cells

7 - Cardiac dysrhythmias

4 - Hyperkalaemia

6 - Urate nephropathy

5 - Uric acid crystals in urine

2 - Allopurinol (a xanthine oxidase inhibitor) tablets reduce urate formation

1 - Correction of dehydration by normal saline solution I.V.

3 - Complications are reduced by alkalinisation of urine

Maintenance chemotherapy is essential following achievement of remission and appears to require at least two drugs, (usually methotrexate and 6-mercaptopurine), continued for at least two years. The child is assessed monthly with a blood count.

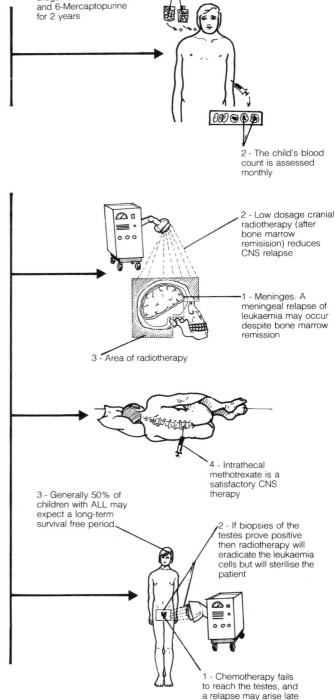

1 - Maintenance therapy requires 2 drugs — Methotrexate and 6-Mercaptopurine for 2 years

2 - The child's blood count is assessed monthly

It has been recognised for some time that the systemic chemotherapy just described does not penetrate the CNS and that meningeal relapse of leukaemia may occur in the face of systemic/bone marrow remission. It is now routine to deliver CNS therapy with intrathecal methotrexate and one course of low dose cranial radiotherapy once the bone marrow is in remission, and such therapy has dramatically reduced the incidence of CNS relapse. In males, the testes also appear to be sites where chemotherapy fails to reach and testicular relapse is also recognised as a late site for solitary relapse. Prophylactic therapy to the testes is not routinely given, but screening testicular biopsies are recommended and, if positive, radiotherapy will eradicate the leukaemia cells here, (but regrettably sterilise the patient also).

2 - Low dosage cranial radiotherapy (after bone marrow remisision) reduces CNS relapse

1 - Meninges. A meningeal relapse of leukaemia may occur despite bone marrow remission

3 - Area of radiotherapy

4 - Intrathecal methotrexate is a satisfactory CNS therapy

3 - Generally 50% of children with ALL may expect a long-term survival free period

2 - If biopsies of the testes prove positive then radiotherapy will eradicate the leukaemia cells but will sterilise the patient

Overall, nearly 50% of all children with ALL may expect long-term disease free survival. Adult patients with ALL are treated similarly but have a slightly less favourable outcome.

1 - Chemotherapy fails to reach the testes, and a relapse may arise late from this site

74

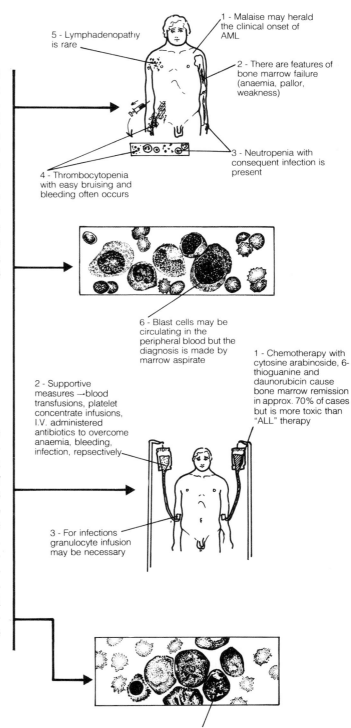

5 - Lymphadenopathy is rare

1 - Malaise may herald the clinical onset of AML

2 - There are features of bone marrow failure (anaemia, pallor, weakness)

3 - Neutropenia with consequent infection is present

4 - Thrombocytopenia with easy bruising and bleeding often occurs

Acute Myeloblastic Leukaemia (AML)

– AML occurs mainly in adults with an incidence considerably less than the common adult cancers (eg. bronchus and breast cancer). The clinical onset may be non-specific with malaise but usually there are the features of bone marrow failure; anaemia (with pallor, weakness, dyspnoea etc.) neutropenia (with infections), and thrombocytopenia (with easy bruising and bleeding). Blast cells may be circulating in the peripheral blood but the more certain diagnosis is made by a marrow aspirate. Lymphadenopathy is unusual in AML.

6 - Blast cells may be circulating in the peripheral blood but the diagnosis is made by marrow aspirate

1 - Chemotherapy with cytosine arabinoside, 6-thioguanine and daunorubicin cause bone marrow remission in approx. 70% of cases but is more toxic than "ALL" therapy

2 - Supportive measures —-blood transfusions, platelet concentrate infusions, I.V. administered antibiotics to overcome anaemia, bleeding, infection, repsectively

Induction chemotherapy with cytosine arabinoside, 6-thioguanine and daunorubicin results in bone marrow remission in approximately 70% of cases. The drug therapy required to achieve remission is considerably more myelotoxic than ALL therapy and these patients require acute nursing care and supportive measures. Thus blood transfusions, platelet concentrate infusions and intravenous combinations of antibiotics are frequently necessary to overcome anaemia, bleeding and infection during therapy. During infections, granulocyte infusions may also be needed.

3 - For infections granulocyte infusion may be necessary

4 - Blast Cells

Unlike ALL, it has proved extremely difficult to maintain bone marrow remission in AML and most patients relapse and die within 3 years of diagnosis. Recently, high dose, whole body radiation to a dose beyond 'marrow death', and then rescue with a bone marrow transplant has shown early promise as a means of eradicating 'the last leukaemic cell', but the method is still very much a procedure for specialist centres.

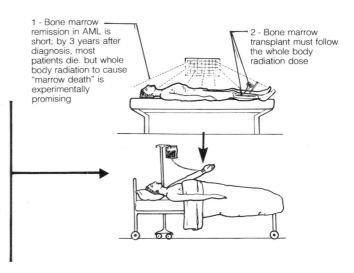

1 - Bone marrow remission in AML is short; by 3 years after diagnosis, most patients die. but whole body radiation to cause "marrow death" is experimentally promising

2 - Bone marrow transplant must follow the whole body radiation dose

Chronic Myeloid Leukaemia (CML) – This unusual form of leukaemia usually afflicts middle aged adults, being slightly more common in males. The clinical onset is insidious with tiredness and symptoms of anaemia being most prominent. There is frequently large or massive hepatosplenomegaly which may cause abdominal discomfort. The typical blood count shows anaemia with a high, sometimes very high (eg. 300×10^9/l) white count largely comprised of the more differentiated forms of the myeloid series, (promyelocytes, myelocytes, metamyelocytes, neutrophils). Although the diagnosis may already seem likely, a bone marrow examination is useful and a low neutrophil alkaline phosphatase helps differentiate CML from a 'leukaemoid reaction'.

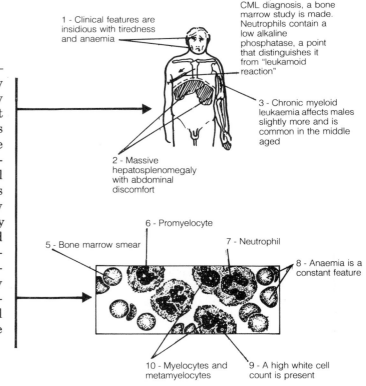

1 - Clinical features are insidious with tiredness and anaemia

4 - Despite obvious CML diagnosis, a bone marrow study is made. Neutrophils contain a low alkaline phosphatase, a point that distinguishes it from "leukamoid reaction"

3 - Chronic myeloid leukaemia affects males slightly more and is common in the middle aged

2 - Massive hepatosplenomegaly with abdominal discomfort

5 - Bone marrow smear

6 - Promyelocyte

7 - Neutrophil

8 - Anaemia is a constant feature

10 - Myelocytes and metamyelocytes

9 - A high white cell count is present

The bone marrow will also assist in diagnosing a blast transformation (see below). There is also a well recognised cytogenetic association with CML cells; this comprises the loss of a variable quantity of genetic material from the long arm of chromosome 22, (the Philadelphia chromosome); this is also of diagnostic use.

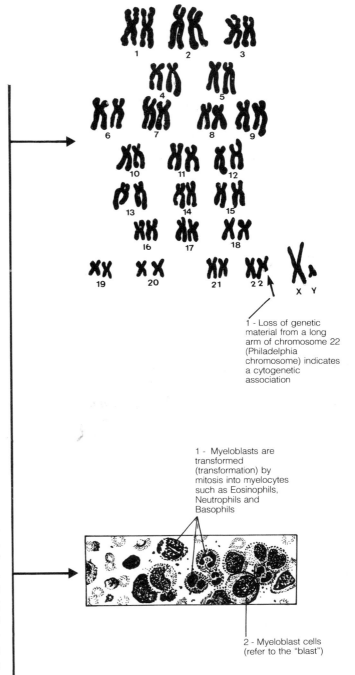

1 - Loss of genetic material from a long arm of chromosome 22 (Philadelphia chromosome) indicates a cytogenetic association

1 - Myeloblasts are transformed (transformation) by mitosis into myelocytes such as Eosinophils, Neutrophils and Basophils

2 - Myeloblast cells (refer to the "blast")

The clinical course of CML comprises an initial chronic phase and a subsequent phase of blast transformation (blast crisis). The patient usually presents in the chronic phase and remission is usually achieved with busulphan, (an orally active, alkylating agent). The drug is given a 0.06mg/kg daily (up to 4mg daily) until the white count falls below $25 \times 10^9/l$ or thrombocytopenia occurs, and initiation of therapy is covered by allopurinol (see above). Maintenance doses of the drug titrate the leukaemic count/cell mass against the potentially serious myelosuppresive action of busulphan. Splenic radiotherapy has a limited therapeutic role in selected patients.

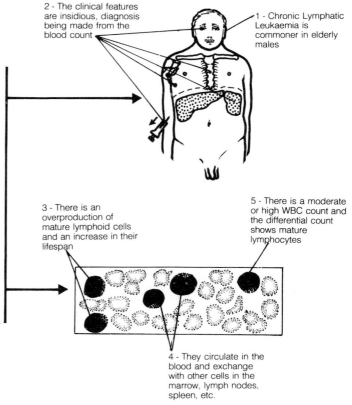

4 - WBC count falls with therapy

3 - Thrombocytopenia occurs

2 - Remission by Busulphan, an orally active alkylating agent in doses of 0.06mg/kg – 4mg daily till WBC falls to 25×10^9/l

5 - The initial therapy is covered by allopurinol

1 - The patient usually presents in the chronic phase

The majority of patients benefit from such therapy for two or three years but a blast transformation usually occurs at some stage with death in a chemoresistant form of AML. Bone marrow transplantation also has a role in CML.

6 - Splenic radiotherapy is used in only a few patients. Most therapies are helpful but blast transformation and chemoresistancy results in death in 2 or 3 years

2 - The clinical features are insidious, diagnosis being made from the blood count

1 - Chronic Lymphatic Leukaemia is commoner in elderly males

Chronic Lymphatic Leukaemia (CLL) – CLL is a more common form of leukaemia than CML and is mostly encountered in the elderly, being uncommon in people less than 45 years; it is commoner in males. In CLL, there is an overproduction of mature lymphoid cells, the life span of which is prolonged; they circulate in the blood and exchange with others in the marrow, lymph nodes, spleen etc. The clinical onset is usually extremely insidious and the diagnosis may be made incidentally on a routine peripheral blood count; the peripheral blood white count may be modestly elevated or very high (eg. 100-200 $\times$ 10^9/l) and the differential shows mature lymphocytes.

3 - There is an overproduction of mature lymphoid cells and an increase in their lifespan

5 - There is a moderate or high WBC count and the differential count shows mature lymphocytes

4 - They circulate in the blood and exchange with other cells in the marrow, lymph nodes, spleen, etc.

Later, lymphadenopathy may call the patient to medical attention, or anaemia – the anaemia being bue to marrow compromise, or occasionally to Coombs' positive haemolysis.

CLL shows a very variable progression after diagnosis and it is worth emphasising that although it is chemo-sensitive initially, it is never chemo-curable. In some patients with a low presenting white count and few clinical symptoms, it may be justifiable to observe the patient off all therapy. In patients with symptoms due to a larger tumour burden (eg. malaise, weight loss associated with lymphadenopathy, hepatosplenomegaly and a high white count), then chemotherapy is indicated. Indeed, all patients with white counts in excess of $100 \times 10^9/l$ will benefit from therapy. The orally active alkylating agent chlorambucil (eg. 8mg/m^2 daily $\times$ 10, repeated monthly after a routine blood count and clinical review) is as effective as any other therapy, although prednisolone is also useful where there is myelosuppression or haemolysis. Painful lymph node masses that fail to respond to chemotherapy respond well to radiotherapy.

Although some patients live for a long time with CLL, the median survival for the disease is approximately four years.

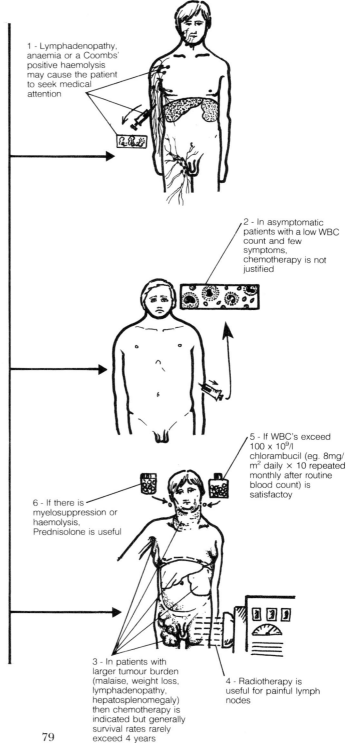

1 - Lymphadenopathy, anaemia or a Coombs' positive haemolysis may cause the patient to seek medical attention

2 - In asymptomatic patients with a low WBC count and few symptoms, chemotherapy is not justified

5 - If WBC's exceed $100 \times 10^9/l$ chlorambucil (eg. 8mg/m^2 daily $\times$ 10 repeated monthly after routine blood count) is satisfactoy

6 - If there is myelosuppression or haemolysis, Prednisolone is useful

3 - In patients with larger tumour burden (malaise, weight loss, lymphadenopathy, hepatosplenomegaly) then chemotherapy is indicated but generally survival rates rarely exceed 4 years

4 - Radiotherapy is useful for painful lymph nodes

MYELOPROLIFERATIVE DISORDERS

These are a family of malignant diseases arising in the bone marrow and characterised by a proliferation of cells of more than one series, but usually including the megakaryocytes. The disorders usually run a 'chronic' time course ending eventually in marrow failure or blastic transformation. Their cause is unknown.

In myelofibrosis, there is a widespread proliferation of fibroblasts, reticulum cells, and even bone within the red marrow spaces, with obliteration of the red marrow. Marrow cells proliferate in other sites (myeloid metaplasia), such as liver and spleen, and both these organs hypertrophy to large size. Patients are usually elderly and present with symptoms of anaemia or abdominal discomfort due to massive splenomegaly. The blood count almost invariably shows anaemia, (with poikilocytic and nucleated red cells on film), but the platelet count is elevated with a differential suggesting CML. The term 'leuco-erythroblastic anaemia' is used when immature red cells and white cells are seen in the blood film.

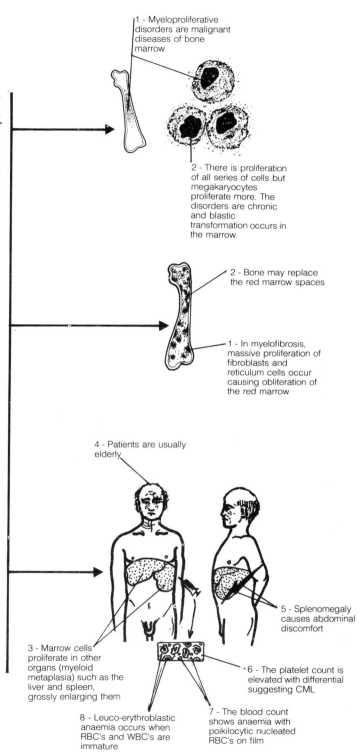

1 - Myeloproliferative disorders are malignant diseases of bone marrow

2 - There is proliferation of all series of cells but megakaryocytes proliferate more. The disorders are chronic and blastic transformation occurs in the marrow

2 - Bone may replace the red marrow spaces

1 - In myelofibrosis, massive proliferation of fibroblasts and reticulum cells occur causing obliteration of the red marrow

4 - Patients are usually elderly

5 - Splenomegaly causes abdominal discomfort

3 - Marrow cells proliferate in other organs (myeloid metaplasia) such as the liver and spleen, grossly enlarging them

6 - The platelet count is elevated with differential suggesting CML

7 - The blood count shows anaemia with poikilocytic nucleated RBC's on film

8 - Leuco-erythroblastic anaemia occurs when RBC's and WBC's are immature

A bone marrow aspirate fails ('dry tap') and a bone trephine shows widespread fibrosis in the marrow with hypocellularity, although megakaryocytes often persist. The serum uric acid is frequently high. There is no satisfactory specific treatment for myelofibrosis, which usually ends in marrow failure within a few years, but allopurinol, folic acid and blood transfusions are appropriate.

Busulphan may have a place in patients with a CML-like picture and splenic ablation may have a limited role where splenic destruction of cells outweighs splenic production of haemopoietic cells. Anabolic steroids have limited efficiency in stimulating red cell recovery.

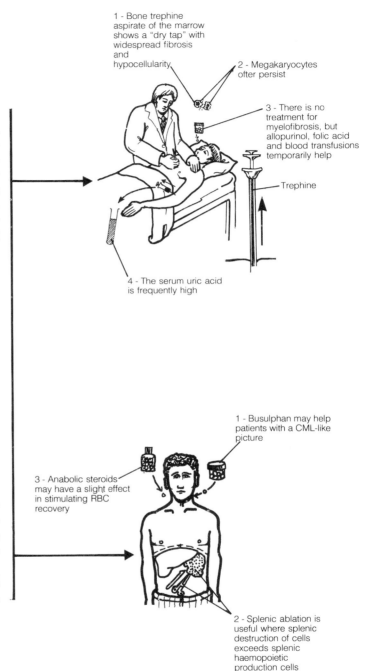

1 - Bone trephine aspirate of the marrow shows a "dry tap" with widespread fibrosis and hypocellularity

2 - Megakaryocytes ofter persist

3 - There is no treatment for myelofibrosis, but allopurinol, folic acid and blood transfusions temporarily help

Trephine

4 - The serum uric acid is frequently high

1 - Busulphan may help patients with a CML-like picture

3 - Anabolic steroids may have a slight effect in stimulating RBC recovery

2 - Splenic ablation is useful where splenic destruction of cells exceeds splenic haemopoietic production cells

In polycythaemia rubra vera (PRV), there is marrow erythroid neoplasia predominantly, together with less marked over production of leucocytes and platelets. PRV tends to affect males beyond middle age and characteristically presents with a blood count of: Hb greater than 18.0 g/dl, RCC greater than 6×10^{12} and PCV greater than 54%. The consequences of this blood picture are blood hyperviscosity with a tendency to thromboses and also an abnormal bleeding tendency, (despite the often elevated platelet count).

1 - In Polycythaemia Rubra Vera there is an erythrocyte neoplasia predominance

2 - Over-production leucocytes and platelets is less marked

3 - Predominant marrow erythroid neoplasia

4 - PRV affect middle-aged males

5 - The Hb is greater than 18·0g/dl; the PCV is greater than 54%

6 - This blood picture causes hyperviscosity, encourages thromboses and abnormal bleeding (despite high platelet count)

The patient with PRV tends to present with headaches or dizziness, tiredness or dyspepsia. On examination, he has a plethoric and cyanosed appearance, is usually hypertensive with distended and engorged retinal veins, (even papilloedema). He will usually have moderate

1 - The patient with PRV suffers dizziness or headaches

2 - Tiredness and dyspepsia are other features. He may be plethoric (distended vessels) and cyanosed

3 - The patient is usually hypertensive

Eye

4 - Papilloedema and engorged retinal veins

hepato-splenomegaly and may be tender in the epigastrium, as PRV is associated with an increased incidence of peptic ulcer. There may be some clinical stigmata of gout. Later in the disease, arterial degenerative disease may lead to cerebrovascular or coronary thromboses. Pruritus is a common symptom in PRV.

The characteristics of the blood count in PRV have been described but the red cells may show stigmata of iron deficiency and these patients are frequently folic acid depleted also. The bone trephine shows hypercellurality including megakaryocyte hyperplasia. The leucocyte alkaline phosphatase score is high and the Philadelphia chromosome negative. The arterial PO_2, and the IVU are both normal — (in contradistintion to most respiratory and renal causes of polycythaemia), and haemoglobin electrophoresis is normal.

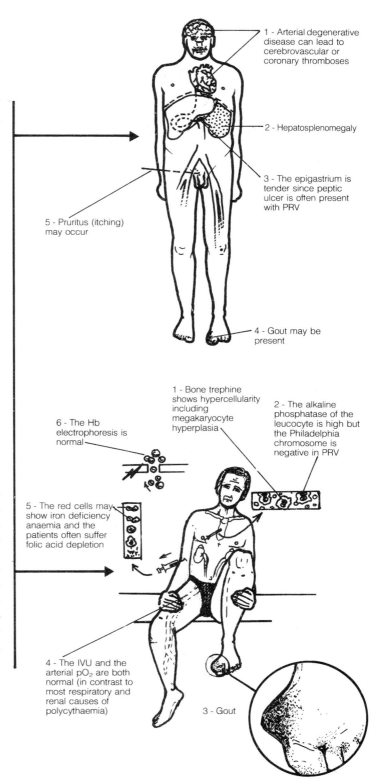

1 - Arterial degenerative disease can lead to cerebrovascular or coronary thromboses

2 - Hepatosplenomegaly

3 - The epigastrium is tender since peptic ulcer is often present with PRV

5 - Pruritus (itching) may occur

4 - Gout may be present

1 - Bone trephine shows hypercellularity including megakaryocyte hyperplasia

2 - The alkaline phosphatase of the leucocyte is high but the Philadelphia chromosome is negative in PRV

6 - The Hb electrophoresis is normal

5 - The red cells may show iron deficiency anaemia and the patients often suffer folic acid depletion

4 - The IVU and the arterial pO_2 are both normal (in contrast to most respiratory and renal causes of polycythaemia)

3 - Gout

There is no cure for PRV but allopurinol, folic acid (and iron) supplements may be important supportive therapy in all patients and cypro-heptadine (a serotonin antagonist) has proved useful for the pruritus. However, the high PCV and its attendant complications usually demand therapy. Phlebotomies (250-500ml) should be performed every few days until the PCV is down to 45%. Thereafter, many patients may be managed with occasional phlebotomies, although every patient is assessed monthly with a blood count.

Where the phlebotomies are required very frequently or in patients with uncomfortable splenomegaly or a high platelet count, then myelosuppressive therapy is indicated. This will apply to most patients over the age of 40 years. ^{32}Phosphorus is a ß emitting isotope that is concentrated in myeloid tissue. An injection of 2.3mCi/m^2, (max 5mCi), usually causes an improvement in the blood count by three months and repeat treatments can be given by a radiotherapist if necessary. Alternatively, an oral alkylating agent (eg. chlorambucil) can be used.

With such therapy, the median survival with PRV is 12 years, but eventual marrow failure or leukaemic transformation occur in most patients and prove fatal.

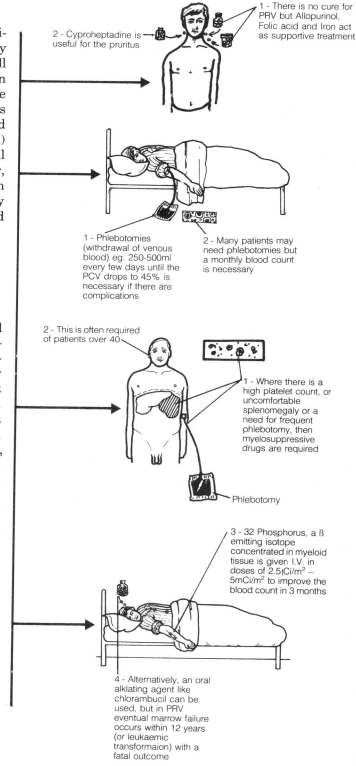

2 - Cyproheptadine is useful for the pruritus

1 - There is no cure for PRV but Allopurinol, Folic acid and Iron act as supportive treatment

1 - Phlebotomies (withdrawal of venous blood) eg. 250-500ml every few days until the PCV drops to 45% is necessary if there are complications

2 - Many patients may need phlebotomies but a monthly blood count is necessary

2 - This is often required of patients over 40

1 - Where there is a high platelet count, or uncomfortable splenomegaly or a need for frequent phlebotomy, then myelosuppressive drugs are required

Phlebotomy

3 - 32 Phosphorus, a ß emitting isotope concentrated in myeloid tissue is given I.V. in doses of 2.5|Ci/m^2 – 5mCi/m^2 to improve the blood count in 3 months

4 - Alternatively, an oral alklating agent like chlorambucil can be used, but in PRV eventual marrow failure occurs within 12 years (or leukaemic transformaion) with a fatal outcome

THE LYMPHOMAS

Hodgkin's Disease (H.D.) – H.D. is a malignant condition of lymphatic tissue that most commonly afflicts young adults, although the condition may occur in children and older adults.

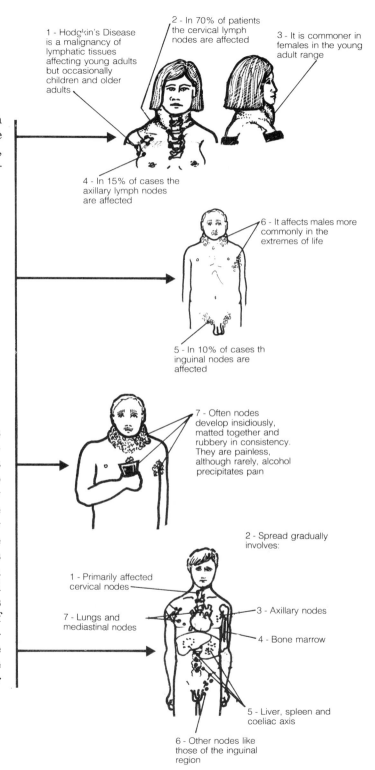

1 - Hodgkin's Disease is a malignancy of lymphatic tissues affecting young adults but occasionally children and older adults

2 - In 70% of patients the cervical lymph nodes are affected

3 - It is commoner in females in the young adult range

4 - In 15% of cases the axillary lymph nodes are affected

6 - It affects males more commonly in the extremes of life

5 - In 10% of cases th inguinal nodes are affected

7 - Often nodes develop insidiously, matted together and rubbery in consistency. They are painless, although rarely, alcohol precipitates pain

2 - Spread gradually involves:

1 - Primarily affected cervical nodes

3 - Axillary nodes

4 - Bone marrow

7 - Lungs and mediastinal nodes

5 - Liver, spleen and coeliac axis

6 - Other nodes like those of the inguinal region

It is commoner in males at the extremes of life, whereas there is a slight predominance of females in the young adult population. Hodgkin's disease seems to arise in one focus and in approximately 70% of patients cervical lymph nodes are affected. In 15% of patients the axillary nodes and in 10% the inguinal nodes are the first affected glands. Often the nodes develop insidiously and are rubbery in consistency and frequently matted together; they are usually painless although the extra-ordinary symptom of pain in the nodes after alcohol is well-recognised although rare. The disease tends to spread to contiguous lymph node groups before it metastasises further afield. Mediastinal node involvement and then infradiaphragmatic spread (particularly to the spleen and coelic axis nodes) commonly follow the cervical presentations. Eventually, systemic manifestations develop – malaise, weight loss, fever, pruritus. Untreated, the disease is fatal.

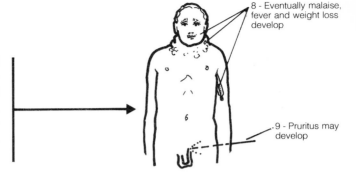

8 - Eventually malaise, fever and weight loss develop

9 - Pruritus may develop

Lymph node biopsy provides the histological diagnosis – the typical picture being of effaced lymph node architecture due to a mixture of lymphocytes and abnormal reticulum cells, (especially the characteristic Reed-Sternberg cells), plus other cells including eosinophils. There are four histological subgroups of H.D. which have prognostic implications: lymphocyte predominant (most favourable), nodular sclerosing, (typically in young adults with mediastinal disease) mixed cellularity and lymphocyte depleted, (least favourable).

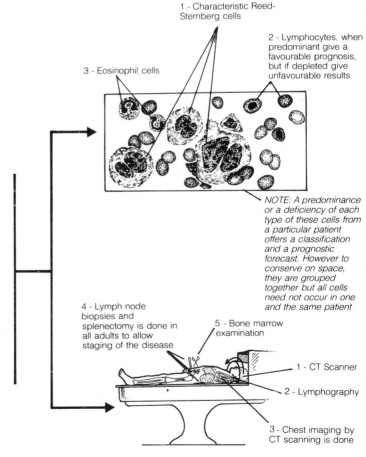

1 - Characteristic Reed-Sternberg cells

2 - Lymphocytes, when predominant give a favourable prognosis, but if depleted give unfavourable results

3 - Eosinophil cells

NOTE: A predominance or a deficiency of each type of these cells from a particular patient offers a classification and a prognostic forecast. However to conserve on space, they are grouped together but all cells need not occur in one and the same patient

4 - Lymph node biopsies and splenectomy is done in all adults to allow staging of the disease

5 - Bone marrow examination

1 - CT Scanner

2 - Lymphography

3 - Chest imaging by CT scanning is done

Of more important significance is the staging of the disease. So important is the accurate assessment of the extent of the dissemination of H.D., that not only are chest imaging (usually C.T. scanning), lymphography and bone marrow examination performed, but also a staging laparotomy with lymph node biopsies and splenectomy is performed in all adults. By such means the patient is grouped as:-

Stage I Disease confined to one lymph node group.

Stage II Disease in more than one lymph node group, but all sites of disease are on one side of the diaphragm.

Stage III Disease in more than one lymph node group on both sides of diaphragm.

Stage IV Extranodal spread, (except small, direct extension of disease out through node capsule).

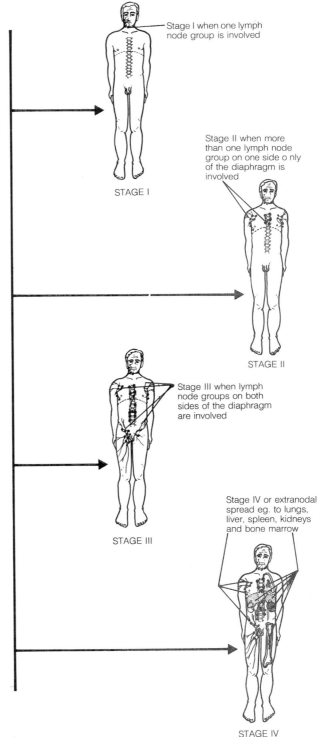

Stage I when one lymph node group is involved

STAGE I

Stage II when more than one lymph node group on one side only of the diaphragm is involved

STAGE II

Stage III when lymph node groups on both sides of the diaphragm are involved

STAGE III

Stage IV or extranodal spread eg. to lungs, liver, spleen, kidneys and bone marrow

STAGE IV

Lastly, these four stages (Ann Arbor stages) may be suffixed A or B depending on whether the patient has systemic symptoms; (the relevant 'B' determining symptoms being: drenching night sweats, 10% of body weight loss in last 6 months and fever to more than 37.5°C for more than 3 days in one week). Thus one might conclude that a patient has stage I_A or II_B or IV_A disease etc.

The accuracy of staging and treatment at a centre specialising in radiotherapy and oncology is stressed here because H.D. is a curable disease but treatment methods differ with staging. There is no doubt that the optimal management of stage I_A – II_A disease is with modern megavoltage radiotherapy administered by specialists. Small bulk III_A disease is also curable by radiotherapy, all the radiation techniques encompassing lymph nodes contiguous to the involved ones. For suffix 'B' diseases and stage IV cases a majority of patients are still curable with a well-established four drug combination (mustine, vincristine, procarbazine, prednisolone), and this chemotherapy is also appropriate for any patient who relapses after radiotherapy.

Overall, two-thirds of patients with H.D. may expect cure and a higher fraction of early stage patients. Cure rates are higher in specialist centres.

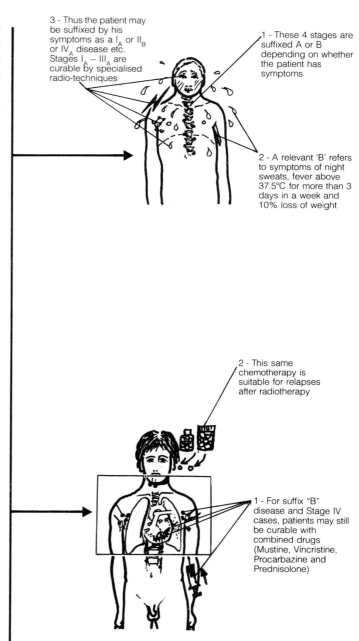

3 - Thus the patient may be suffixed by his symptoms as a I_A or II_B or IV_A disease etc. Stages I_A – III_A are curable by specialised radio-techniques

1 - These 4 stages are suffixed A or B depending on whether the patient has symptoms

2 - A relevant 'B' refers to symptoms of night sweats, fever above 37.5°C for more than 3 days in a week and 10% loss of weight

2 - This same chemotherapy is suitable for relapses after radiotherapy

1 - For suffix "B" disease and Stage IV cases, patients may still be curable with combined drugs (Mustine, Vincristine, Procarbazine and Prednisolone)

Non-Hodgkin Lymphomas (NHL) – This heterogenous collection of lymphoid malignancies may present, (like Hodgkin's disease), with lymphadenopathy confined to one lymph node group, or they may present with rapidly progressive disease infiltrating bone marrow and other organs and proving fatal. Not infrequently, large presenting primary masses in chest or abdomen occur together with metastases. The histological classification of NHL is one of the most controversial in oncology. In summary, 'low grade' histology and follicular architecture in the affected nodes are good prognostic indicators, whereas diffuse effacement of the nodes by a sheet of blast-like cells, (diffuse architecture termed 'high grade' by the histologist), represents poor prognostic NHL.

Although the previously described Ann Arbor staging system is used to assess NHL, the pattern or spread in NHL is less predictable than in H.D. and the initial investigative work-up of these patients does not demand a laparotomy.

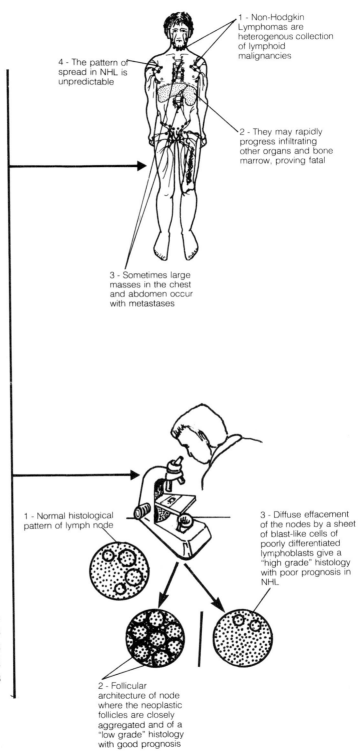

4 - The pattern of spread in NHL is unpredictable

1 - Non-Hodgkin Lymphomas are heterogenous collection of lymphoid malignancies

2 - They may rapidly progress infiltrating other organs and bone marrow, proving fatal

3 - Sometimes large masses in the chest and abdomen occur with metastases

1 - Normal histological pattern of lymph node

3 - Diffuse effacement of the nodes by a sheet of blast-like cells of poorly differentiated lymphoblasts give a "high grade" histology with poor prognosis in NHL

2 - Follicular architecture of node where the neoplastic follicles are closely aggregated and of a "low grade" histology with good prognosis

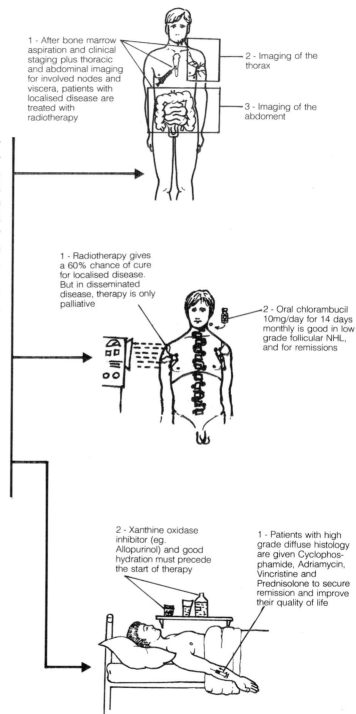

1 - After bone marrow aspiration and clinical staging plus thoracic and abdominal imaging for involved nodes and viscera, patients with localised disease are treated with radiotherapy

2 - Imaging of the thorax

3 - Imaging of the abdoment

1 - Radiotherapy gives a 60% chance of cure for localised disease. But in disseminated disease, therapy is only palliative

2 - Oral chlorambucil 10mg/day for 14 days monthly is good in low grade follicular NHL, and for remissions

2 - Xanthine oxidase inhibitor (eg. Allopurinol) and good hydration must precede the start of therapy

1 - Patients with high grade diffuse histology are given Cyclophosphamide, Adriamycin, Vincristine and Prednisolone to secure remission and improve their quality of life

After clinical staging with bone marrow aspiration and thoracic and abdominal imaging for involved nodes or viscera, patients with localised disease are treated by radiotherapy and stand a 60% chance of cure whilst those with disseminated disease can be well-palliated (often for years) with chemotherapy, although this is rarely curative. In summary, oral chlorambucil (10mg daily × 14, repeated monthly), used alone is as good as any other regime for low grade follicular NHL and lengthy remissions occur. Those patients with high grade, diffuse histology require intensive drug regimes (usually including cyclophosphamide, adriamycin, vincristine, prednisolone) to achieve a remission and this is usually achieved with a worthwhile improvement in the quality of life, but may be of short duration. As in leukaemia therapy, good hydration and xanthine oxidase inhibition (with allopurinol) must always precede initiation of therapy.

In children, most NHL is of the high grade type with a high propensity to early spread. Intensive chemotherapy has had success in early stage disease and cure is possible. One particular childhood NHL, Burkitt lymphoma, exemplifies this rapid growth and dissemination pattern, (with frequent early bone marrow and CSF involvement). Burkitt lymphoma occurs particularly in children aged 2-14 years in tropical Africa. They present with facial (40%) or abdominal (40%) swellings and quickly become very ill due to rapidly progressing disease. The disease rapidly responds to combination chemotherapy with a chance of cure in early stage disease; unfortunately, the disease is frequently advanced at presentation and chemotherapy is only able to temporarily palliate.

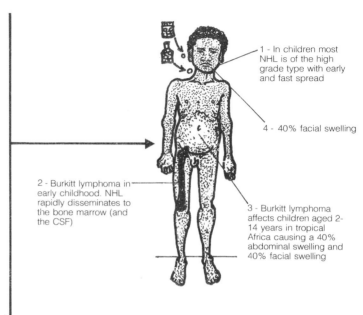

1 - In children most NHL is of the high grade type with early and fast spread

4 - 40% facial swelling

2 - Burkitt lymphoma in early childhood. NHL rapidly disseminates to the bone marrow (and the CSF)

3 - Burkitt lymphoma affects children aged 2-14 years in tropical Africa causing a 40% abdominal swelling and 40% facial swelling

MULTIPLE MYELOMA

Multiple myeloma is a bone marrow neoplasm caused by a malignant proliferation of plasma cells; the malignancy arises from a single clone of plasma cells and when these 'function', they all produce an identical immunoglobulin or immunoglobulin fragment, (monoclonal protein, M-protein, paraprotein) detectable

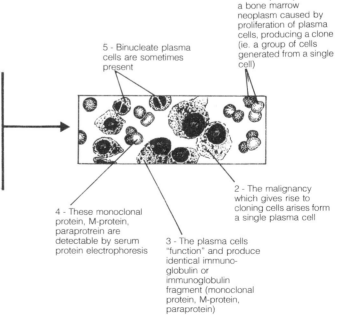

1 - Multiple myeloma is a bone marrow neoplasm caused by proliferation of plasma cells, producing a clone (ie. a group of cells generated from a single cell)

5 - Binucleate plasma cells are sometimes present

2 - The malignancy which gives rise to cloning cells arises form a single plasma cell

4 - These monoclonal protein, M-protein, paraprotrein are detectable by serum protein electrophoresis

3 - The plasma cells "function" and produce identical immuno-globulin or immunoglobulin fragment (monoclonal protein, M-protein, paraprotein)

by serum protein electrophoresis. In addition, excessive production and secretion of immunoglobulin light chain fragments (kappa or lambda) may occur; these light chain protein molecules are detectable in the urine, (Bence Jones Protein, BJP) where they are of diagnostic importance. The diffuse marrow infiltration with patchy, often well-circumscribed areas of lysis of the overlying bone cortex account for the anaemia (or pancycytopenia) and the weakened bones encountered in this condition. The paraprotein production (most commonly IgG-55%, then IgA-25%, BJP only 12%) occurs at the expense of normal immunoglobulin, whose synthesis is often much reduced, (immune paresis), rendering the patient more liable to infection; furthermore, the paraproteinaemia may also be toxic to the renal tubules and renal failure may occur.

The clinical picture usually has an insidious onset. Almost sixty per cent of patients suffer from bone pain and many patients present with symptoms of anaemia or uraemia. Bacterial infections are also common and may be serious. Physical examination may not disclose any diagnostic clues and lymphadenopathy is not a feature of myeloma.

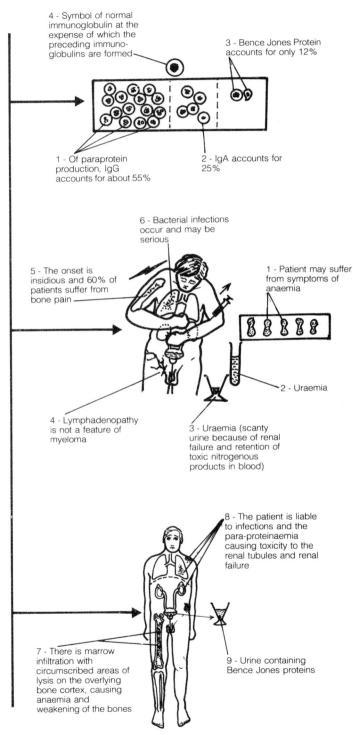

4 - Symbol of normal immunoglobulin at the expense of which the preceding immuno-globulins are formed

3 - Bence Jones Protein accounts for only 12%

1 - Of paraprotein production, IgG accounts for about 55%

2 - IgA accounts for 25%

6 - Bacterial infections occur and may be serious

5 - The onset is insidious and 60% of patients suffer from bone pain

1 - Patient may suffer from symptoms of anaemia

2 - Uraemia

4 - Lymphadenopathy is not a feature of myeloma

3 - Uraemia (scanty urine because of renal failure and retention of toxic nitrogenous products in blood)

8 - The patient is liable to infections and the para-proteinaemia causing toxicity to the renal tubules and renal failure

7 - There is marrow infiltration with circumscribed areas of lysis on the overlying bone cortex, causing anaemia and weakening of the bones

9 - Urine containing Bence Jones proteins

The diagnosis is suggested by a very high ESR and rouleaux formation on the blood smear, (both reflecting a high paraprotein level). Typical X-ray appearances are multiple, well-circumscribed or 'punched-out' lytic bone lesions classically in the calvarium of the skull, ribs and axial skeleton. The serum electrophoretic strip classically demonstrates a monoclonal paraprotein of greater than 30g/l with immune paresis, and BJP may be present in the urine. The bone marrow aspirate gives the diagnosis when it shows excessive numbers of malignant plasma cells. Interestingly, the lytic bone lesions do not engender a surrounding osteoblastic reaction and thus bone scanning and alkaline phosphatase levels underestimate the extent of disease.

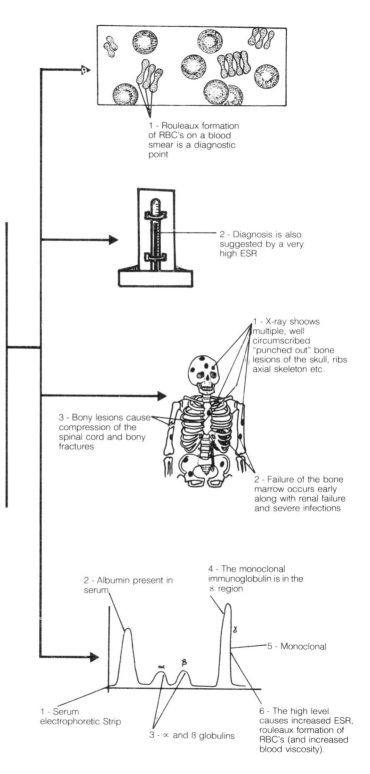

1 - Rouleaux formation of RBC's on a blood smear is a diagnostic point

2 - Diagnosis is also suggested by a very high ESR

1 - X-ray shoows multiple, well circumscribed "punched out" bone lesions of the skull, ribs axial skeleton etc.

3 - Bony lesions cause compression of the spinal cord and bony fractures

2 - Failure of the bone marrow occurs early along with renal failure and severe infections

2 - Albumin present in serum

4 - The monoclonal immunoglobulin is in the ɣ region

5 - Monoclonal

1 - Serum electrophoretic Strip

3 - ∝ and ß globulins

6 - The high level causes increased ESR, rouleaux formation of RBC's (and increased blood viscosity).

The major complications of myeloma are pathological fractures in bones or spinal cord compression due to vertebral collapse, bone marrow failure, severe infections and renal failure. In addition, hypercalcaemia, hyperuricaemia and hyperviscosity may occur in this condition and exacerbate the renal failure. Amyloidosis may occur secondary to myeloma and may also exacerbate uraemia.

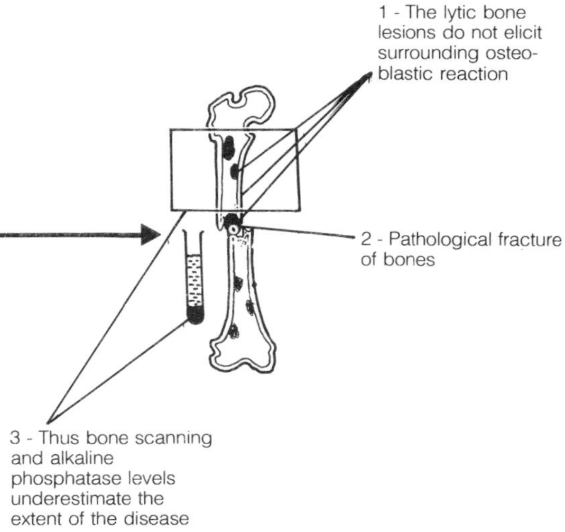

1 - The lytic bone lesions do not elicit surrounding osteoblastic reaction

2 - Pathological fracture of bones

3 - Thus bone scanning and alkaline phosphatase levels underestimate the extent of the disease

4 - Bone pain and lytic lesion in the cortices of long bones should be irradiated to prevent fractures

1 - Amyloidosis follows myeloma and may exacerbate uraemia

Local sites of bone pain are best controlled by radiotherapy and lytic lesions in the cortices of long bones should also be irradiated to prevent pathological fractures.

2 - Hypercalaemia

3 - Hyperuricaemia

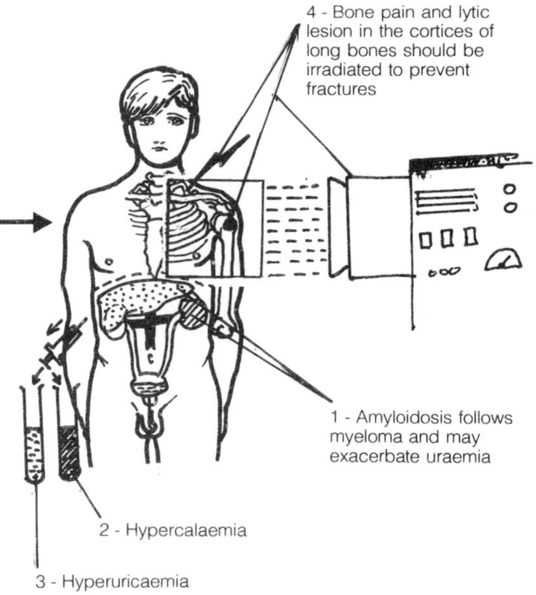

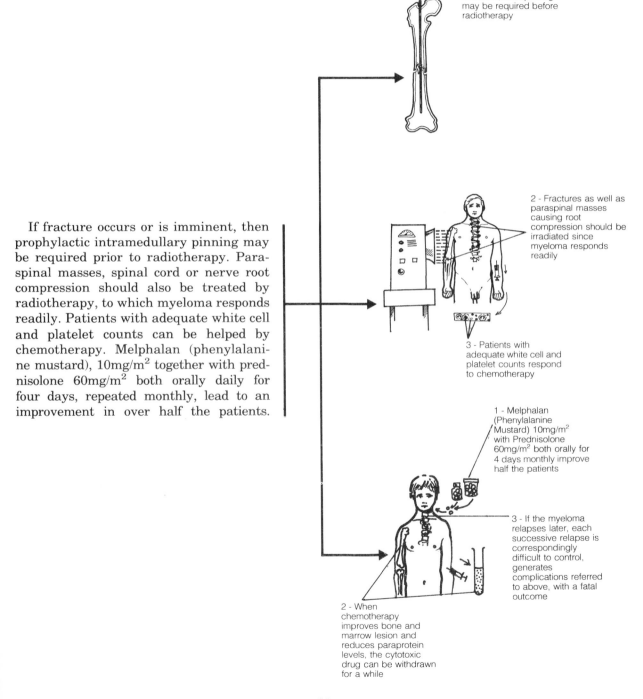

1 - If the fracture seems imminent, then pinning may be required before radiotherapy

2 - Fractures as well as paraspinal masses causing root compression should be irradiated since myeloma responds readily

3 - Patients with adequate white cell and platelet counts respond to chemotherapy

1 - Melphalan (Phenylalanine Mustard) 10mg/m^2 with Prednisolone 60mg/m^2 both orally for 4 days monthly improve half the patients

3 - If the myeloma relapses later, each successive relapse is correspondingly difficult to control, generates complications referred to above, with a fatal outcome

2 - When chemotherapy improves bone and marrow lesion and reduces paraprotein levels, the cytotoxic drug can be withdrawn for a while

If fracture occurs or is imminent, then prophylactic intramedullary pinning may be required prior to radiotherapy. Paraspinal masses, spinal cord or nerve root compression should also be treated by radiotherapy, to which myeloma responds readily. Patients with adequate white cell and platelet counts can be helped by chemotherapy. Melphalan (phenylalanine mustard), 10mg/m^2 together with prednisolone 60mg/m^2 both orally daily for four days, repeated monthly, lead to an improvement in over half the patients.

When the patient has achieved his maximal improvement on the chemotherapy, (no new bone lesion, stable bone marrow, stable and reduced paraprotein levels), it is often possible to withdraw the cytotoxic therapy for a while. However, the myeloma relapses again after a variable interval and proves more difficult to control again with each relapse; it is eventually lethal either due to one of the complications listed above, or due to a terminal 'acute leukaemia' phase.

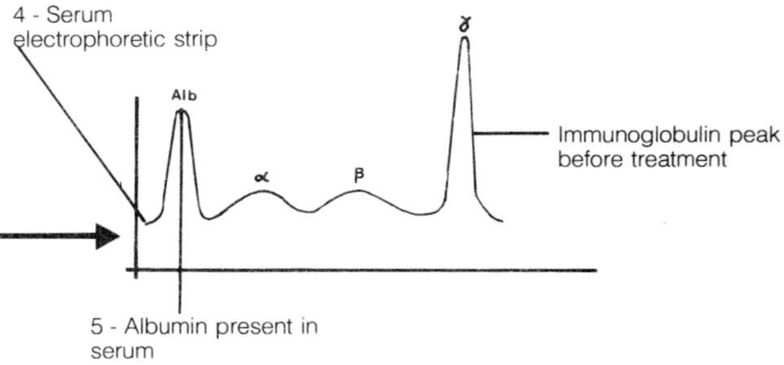

4 - Serum electrophoretic strip

Alb

α   β   γ

Immunoglobulin peak before treatment

5 - Albumin present in serum

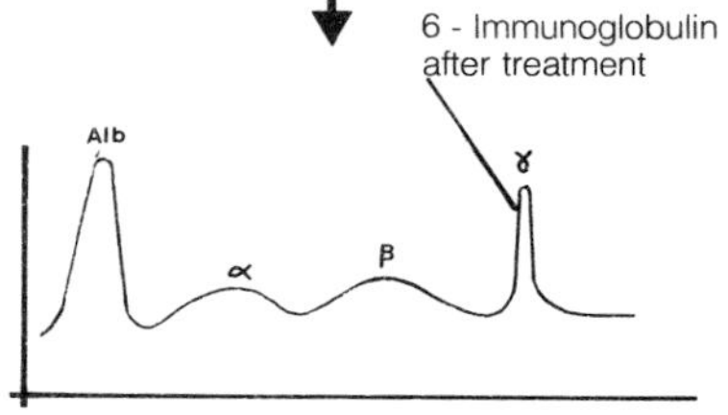

6 - Immunoglobulin after treatment

Alb

α   β   γ

Other essential treatment for myeloma will often include analgesics, blood transfusions and prolonged courses of antibiotics. Adequate hydration and corticosteroids are both important in the management of hypercalcaemia.

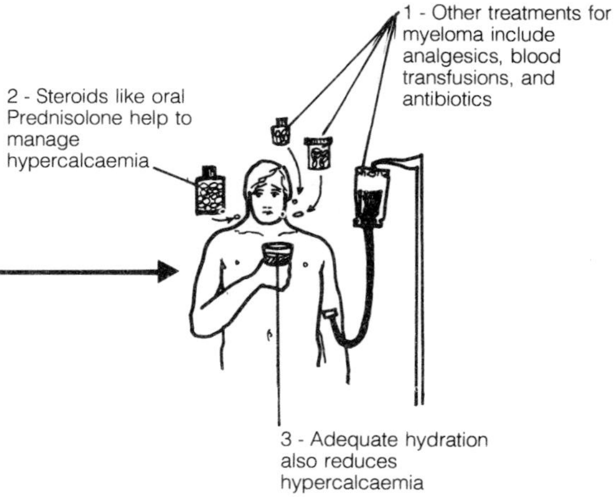

1 - Other treatments for myeloma include analgesics, blood transfusions, and antibiotics

2 - Steroids like oral Prednisolone help to manage hypercalcaemia

3 - Adequate hydration also reduces hypercalcaemia

Benign monoclonal gammopathy and localised plasmacytoma – Two conditions may be confused with or precede myeloma.

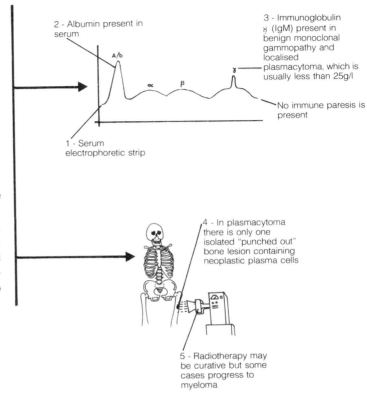

2 - Albumin present in serum

3 - Immunoglobulin ɤ (IgM) present in benign monoclonal gammopathy and localised plasmacytoma, which is usually less than 25g/l

No immune paresis is present

1 - Serum electrophoretic strip

In benign monoclonal gammopathy, there is a monoclonal protein demonstrable on serum protein electrophoresis, (usually less than 25g/l), but no bone cortex or marrow abnormalities nor immune paresis. In localised plasmacytoma, there appears one isolated 'punched-out', lytic bone lesion containing neoplastic plasma cells. Radiotherapy may be curative although some cases progress to myeloma.

4 - In plasmacytoma there is only one isolated "punched out" bone lesion containing neoplastic plasma cells

5 - Radiotherapy may be curative but some cases progress to myeloma

Waldenstrom's Macroglobulinaemia –This condition is often confused with myeloma due to the fact that a paraprotein is present. However, the condition differs from myeloma in that widespread lymphadenopathy and hepatosplenomegaly are common, the Ig secreted is IgM and is attended by hyperviscosity, (with CNS focal and confusional signs – even coma, fundal changes – notably retinal venous suffusion and haemorrhages,

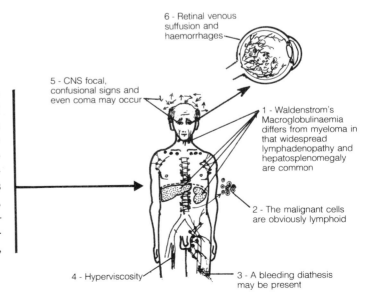

6 - Retinal venous suffusion and haemorrhages

5 - CNS focal, confusional signs and even coma may occur

1 - Waldenstrom's Macroglobulinaemia differs from myeloma in that widespread lymphadenopathy and hepatosplenomegaly are common

2 - The malignant cells are obviously lymphoid

4 - Hyperviscosity

3 - A bleeding diathesis may be present

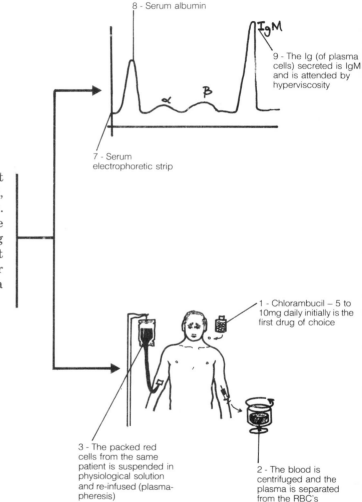

8 - Serum albumin

IgM

9 - The Ig (of plasma cells) secreted is IgM and is attended by hyperviscosity

7 - Serum electrophoretic strip

bleeding diathesis etc.). The malignant cells are usually more obviously lymphoid, (lymphoplasmacytoid) than in myeloma. Although therapy could well be along the lines for myeloma, chlorambucil (5-10 mg daily initially) has become the drug of first choice. The best immediate treatment for the hyperviscosity syndrome is plasma exchange (plasmapheresis).

1 - Chlorambucil – 5 to 10mg daily initially is the first drug of choice

3 - The packed red cells from the same patient is suspended in physiological solution and re-infused (plasma-pheresis)

2 - The blood is centrifuged and the plasma is separated from the RBC's

Immunology

THE IMMUNE RESPONSE

The **immune response** is a tissue reaction (or rather a spectrum of reactions), provoked by the penetration of foreign or mis-recognised proteins (including those in intact organisms e.g. bacteria) – so called antigens (**Ag**), into the systemic circulation or body tissues. Antigens are proteins or glycoproteins (rarely complex carbohydrates). Antigens interact with surface receptors on lymphoid cells (distinguished by surface and functional characteristics into **T** and **B** series).

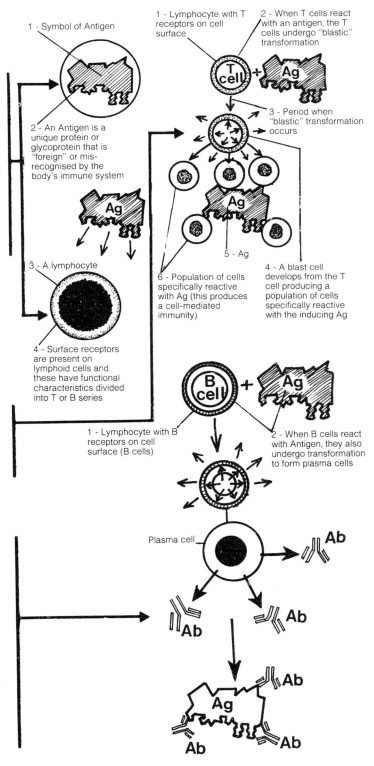

1 - Symbol of Antigen

2 - An Antigen is a unique protein or glycoprotein that is "foreign" or mis-recognised by the body's immune system

3 - A lymphocyte

4 - Surface receptors are present on lymphoid cells and these have functional characteristics divided into T or B series

1 - Lymphocyte with T receptors on cell surface

2 - When T cells react with an antigen, the T cells undergo "blastic" transformation

3 - Period when "blastic" transformation occurs

4 - A blast cell develops from the T cell producing a population of cells specifically reactive with the inducing Ag

5 - Ag

6 - Population of cells specifically reactive with Ag (this produces a cell-mediated immunity)

1 - Lymphocyte with B receptors on cell surface (B cells)

2 - When B cells react with Antigen, they also undergo transformation to form plasma cells

Plasma cell

Following interaction with antigen (activation), **T** cells undergo blastic transformation and cell division producing a progeny population of cells specifically reactive with the inducing **Ag** (**cell-mediated immunity**).

However, when **B** lymphocytes interact with **Ag**, they may differentiate into plasma cells which then secrete a unique protein molecule, called antibody (**Ab**), which avidly binds to the inducing antigen with high specificity. The act of binding (forming the antigen-antibody, **Ag-Ab**, complex), may in itself detoxify an antigen, but more often it facilitates the destruction of the antigen by promoting the phagocytosis of the complex or the destruction of the antigen (e.g. bacterium) by activation of an enzymic cascade of cytocidal effects (e.g. the "complement" cascade) or other events.

This second type of immune reaction is called **humoral immunity.**

Both types of immune reaction share the property that the first encounter with an antigen provokes a slightly delayed and mild reaction, whereas a later reaction provokes a much faster and violent response; it is concluded that an initial encounter (primary immune response), establishes a population of long lived memory cells that can respond more immediately to a secondary encounter. The basis for immunisation against infection is to promote the formation of such long-lived memory cells such that the body is "prepared to fight" the infection, with a secondary immune response.

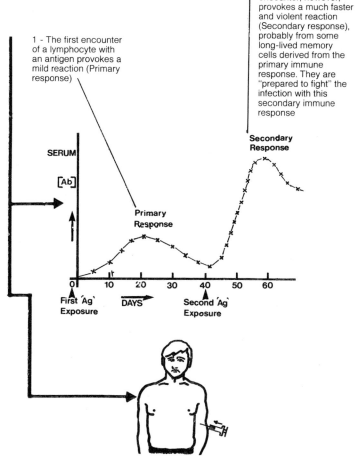

1 - The first encounter of a lymphocyte with an antigen provokes a mild reaction (Primary response)

2 - A later Ab-Ag encounter, however, provokes a much faster and violent reaction (Secondary response), probably from some long-lived memory cells derived from the primary immune response. They are "prepared to fight" the infection with this secondary immune response

Secondary Response

SERUM

[Ab]

Primary Response

First 'Ag' Exposure

DAYS

Second 'Ag' Exposure

The survival value to a host of being able to rid itself of foreign proteins (toxins, infective agents etc.) is obvious. Problems arise, however, when the body mis-recognises normal self-proteins as antigens (e.g. thyroglobulin in **Hashimoto's disease**), and an auto-immune disease results – i.e. the body reacts against its own tissues, possibly destroying them.

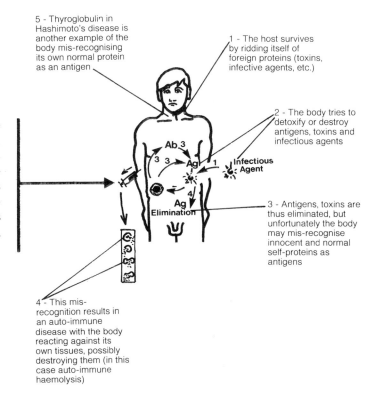

5 - Thyroglobulin in Hashimoto's disease is another example of the body mis-recognising its own normal protein as an antigen

1 - The host survives by ridding itself of foreign proteins (toxins, infective agents, etc.)

2 - The body tries to detoxify or destroy antigens, toxins and infectious agents

3 - Antigens, toxins are thus eliminated, but unfortunately the body may mis-recognise innocent and normal self-proteins as antigens

4 - This mis-recognition results in an auto-immune disease with the body reacting against its own tissues, possibly destroying them (in this case auto-immune haemolysis)

Similarly, problems are encountered in tissue transplantation surgery when subtle differences in tissue antigens between different donor and recipient patients (e.g. blood group **ABO** antigens or the histocompatibility **HLA** derived system of cell antigens) occur and provoke rejection reaction.

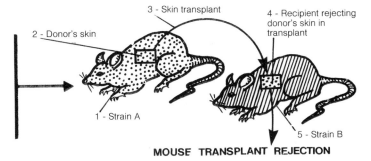

2 - Donor's skin
3 - Skin transplant
4 - Recipient rejecting donor's skin in transplant
1 - Strain A
5 - Strain B

MOUSE TRANSPLANT REJECTION

The **HLA** genes controlling cell surface **Ag** expression are of great interest; there is now known to be an association between several diseases (notably ankylosing spondylitis, Reiter's syndrome, Type I diabetes mellitus, and gluten enteropathy) and the **HLA** phenotype of the individual; this is strong evidence for an immune basis to these particular diseases.

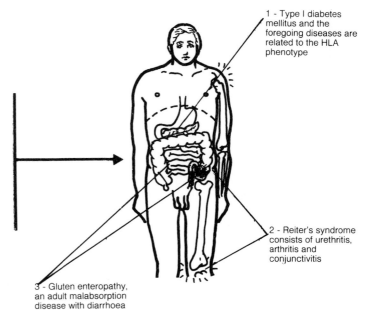

1 - Type I diabetes mellitus and the foregoing diseases are related to the HLA phenotype

2 - Reiter's syndrome consists of urethritis, arthritis and conjunctivitis

3 - Gluten enteropathy, an adult malabsorption disease with diarrhoea

ACTIVATED T CELLS

Following **antigenic stimulation**, there is produced a population of activated **T** lymphocytes capable of specifically killing virally infected host cells, graft cells, tumour cells etc. – all by a cell-mediated immune reaction. The activated **T** lymphocytes carry specific recognition/combining sites on their surface.

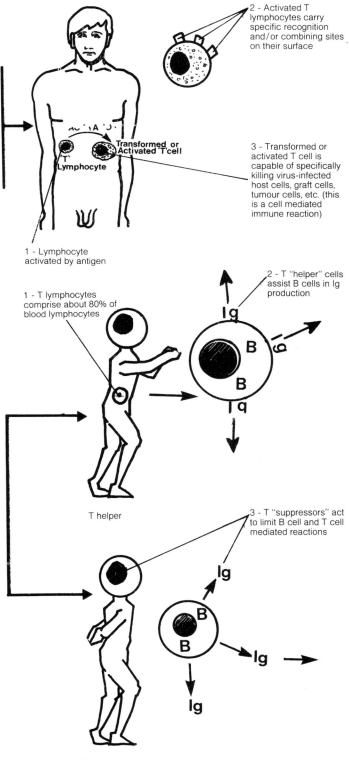

2 - Activated T lymphocytes carry specific recognition and/or combining sites on their surface

Transformed or Activated T cell

3 - Transformed or activated T cell is capable of specifically killing virus-infected host cells, graft cells, tumour cells, etc. (this is a cell mediated immune reaction)

T Lymphocyte

1 - Lymphocyte activated by antigen

1 - T lymphocytes comprise about 80% of blood lymphocytes

2 - T "helper" cells assist B cells in Ig production

Ig

B

B

T helper

3 - T "suppressors" act to limit B cell and T cell mediated reactions

Ig

B

B

Ig

Ig

T suppressor

T lymphocytes comprise approximately 80% of peripheral blood lymphocytes. The discrimination between cell-mediated and humoral immune reactions is too simple and two subsets of **T** lymphocytes are now recognised. **T** "helper" cells assist **B** cells in immunoglobulin production whereas T "suppressor" cells act to limit **B** cell and **T** cell mediated reactions. There are humoral factors which mediate the cross-talk between lymphocytes, macrophages and other cells (lymphokines).

IMMUNOGLOBULINS

Antibodies are proteins of γ-globulin type (immunoglobulins, **Ig**) derived from plasma cells (**B** cell lineage). Each immunoglobulin molecule has two "heavy" and two "light" peptide chains bound together by disulphide bonds and their conformational arrangement allows for the specific antigenic recognition site. The **N**-terminal ends of the molecule are variable in structure allowing for this differing specificity for **Ag**. The **C** terminal ends are constant for the **Ab** class.

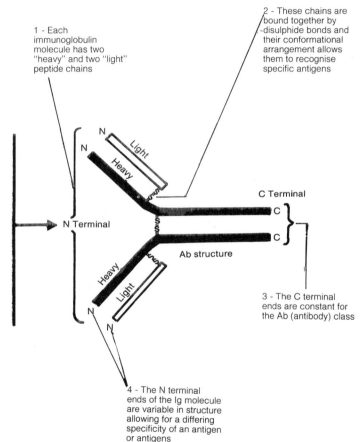

1 - Each immunoglobulin molecule has two "heavy" and two "light" peptide chains

2 - These chains are bound together by disulphide bonds and their conformational arrangement allows them to recognise specific antigens

3 - The C terminal ends are constant for the Ab (antibody) class

4 - The N terminal ends of the Ig molecule are variable in structure allowing for a differing specificity of an antigen or antigens

There are 5 different classes of immuno-globulins (**IgG**, **IgM**, **IgA**, **IgD**, **IgE**). These different classes become important with regard to the different "effector functions" that occur after **Ag-Ab** interaction. For example, **IgG** and **IgM** molecules have sites for complement fixation (and hence activation of the complement cascade) in the F_c section, but **IgD**, **IgA** and **IgE** do not. Only **IgE** has a site for attachment to mast cells (see "Anaphylaxis" below). **IgG** and **IgM** bind to macrophages facilitating pinocytosis of **Ag**, and **IgG** binds to killer (**K**) cells facilitating the so-called antibody dependent cell-mediated cytotoxicity (**ADCC**).

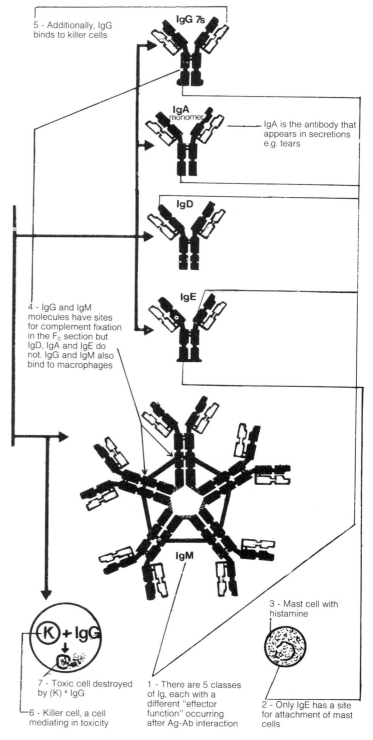

5 - Additionally, IgG binds to killer cells

IgG 7s

IgA monomer

IgA is the antibody that appears in secretions e.g. tears

IgD

4 - IgG and IgM molecules have sites for complement fixation in the F_c section but IgD, IgA and IgE do not. IgG and IgM also bind to macrophages

IgE

IgM

3 - Mast cell with histamine

(K) + IgG

7 - Toxic cell destroyed by (K) ⁴ IgG

6 - Killer cell, a cell mediating in toxicity

1 - There are 5 classes of Ig, each with a different "effector function" occurring after Ag-Ab interaction

2 - Only IgE has a site for attachment of mast cells

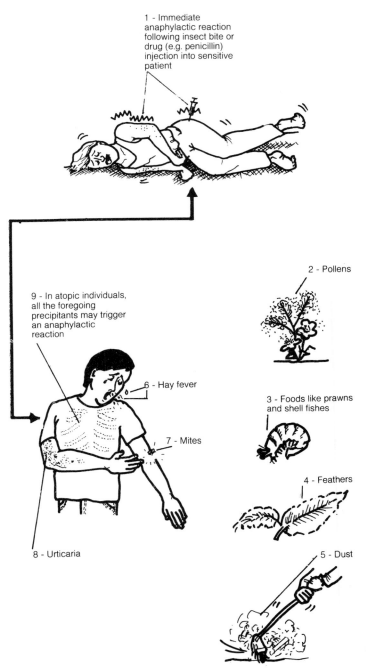

1 - Immediate anaphylactic reaction following insect bite or drug (e.g. penicillin) injection into sensitive patient

COOMBS' AND GEL FOUR TYPES OF HYPERSENSITIVITY
TYPE I - ANAPHYLACTIC SENSITIVITY

In this group of "immediately" occurring reactions can be placed the immediate anaphylactic reactions such as rarely occur following an insect bite or drug (e.g. penicillin) injection into a sensitive individual. This group also includes atopic individuals who are sensitised to foods, pollens, feathers, dust, mites etc. and who manifest their allergy with hay fever, asthma or urticaria.

9 - In atopic individuals, all the foregoing precipitants may trigger an anaphylactic reaction

6 - Hay fever

7 - Mites

8 - Urticaria

2 - Pollens

3 - Foods like prawns and shell fishes

4 - Feathers

5 - Dust

In type I reactivity, the antigen reacts with a specific class of antibody (**IgE**) bound to mast cells or circulating basophils. This **Ag-Ab** interaction triggers the degranulation of the mast cells with release of many pharmacologically active granule constituents (e.g. histamine, serotonin, slow reacting substance etc.).

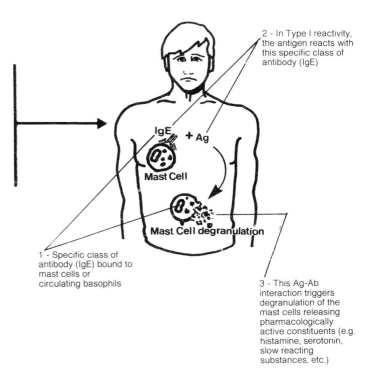

2 - In Type I reactivity, the antigen reacts with this specific class of antibody (IgE)

1 - Specific class of antibody (IgE) bound to mast cells or circulating basophils

3 - This Ag-Ab interaction triggers degranulation of the mast cells releasing pharmacologically active constituents (e.g. histamine, serotonin, slow reacting substances, etc.)

Desensitisation of atopic individuals is possible by multiple small dose injections of the allergens or antigen (**Ag**). The mechanism is sometimes via the induction of **IgG** formation rather than **IgE** production and this may then "block" **Ag-IgE** interactions. Specific therapy is with disodium cromoglycate etc. (see Asthma and Hay Fever sections).

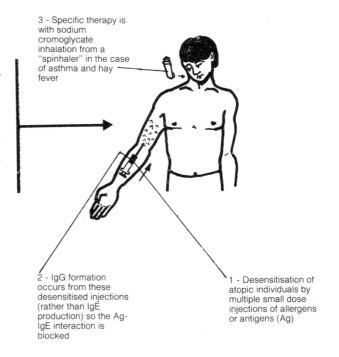

3 - Specific therapy is with sodium cromoglycate inhalation from a "spinhaler" in the case of asthma and hay fever

2 - IgG formation occurs from these desensitised injections (rather than IgE production) so the Ag-IgE interaction is blocked

1 - Desensitisation of atopic individuals by multiple small dose injections of allergens or antigens (Ag)

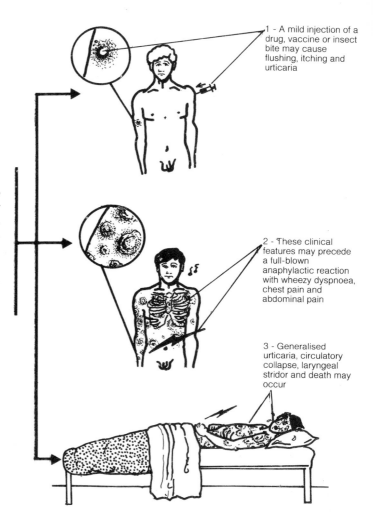

1 - A mild injection of a drug, vaccine or insect bite may cause flushing, itching and urticaria

ANAPHYLACTIC SHOCK

A mild reaction to an injection of a drug, vaccine or insect bite is common with flushing, itching and urticaria (often localised). However, these clinical features may precede a full-blown anaphylactic reaction with wheezy dyspnoea, chest tightness, abdominal pain, generalised urticaria, progressing to circulatory collapse, laryngeal stridor and death.

2 - These clinical features may precede a full-blown anaphylactic reaction with wheezy dyspnoea, chest pain and abdominal pain

3 - Generalised urticaria, circulatory collapse, laryngeal stridor and death may occur

Emergency Management:

1) Adrenaline 1:1000, 0.5ml subcutaneously.
2) Hydrocortisone 200mg i.v. Stat.
3) Diphenhydramine 20mg i.v. Stat (or other antihistamine).
4) Aminophylline 0.5g i.v. over 5 minutes if there is stridor. (Rarely, tracheostomy is required for severe, life-threatening laryngeal stridor.)

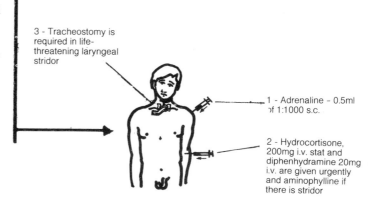

3 - Tracheostomy is required in life-threatening laryngeal stridor

1 - Adrenaline – 0.5ml of 1:1000 s.c.

2 - Hydrocortisone, 200mg i.v. stat and diphenhydramine 20mg i.v. are given urgently and aminophylline if there is stridor

5) Oxygen for cyanosed patients.
6) General measures of circulatory collapse – supine or flat, "tonsillar" position, **CVP** line and colloid infusion.

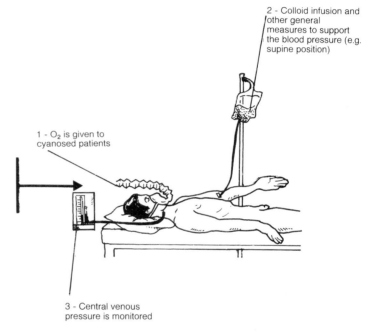

2 - Colloid infusion and other general measures to support the blood pressure (e.g. supine position)

1 - O_2 is given to cyanosed patients

3 - Central venous pressure is monitored

TYPE II - CYTOTOXIC SENSITIVITY

The interaction of **Ab (IgG or IgM)** with a cell surface antigen promotes cell destruction by phagocytosis or direct lysis (particularly via activation of the complement enzymic cascade). Haemolysis as encountered in blood transfusion reactions is one example – blood group **A** patients possess anti **B** cytotoxic antibodies (isohaemagglutinins) and will agglutinate and lyse erythrocytes transfused from a blood group B patient.

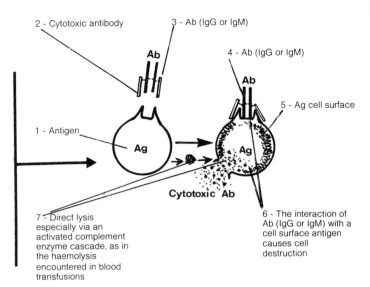

2 - Cytotoxic antibody

3 - Ab (IgG or IgM)

4 - Ab (IgG or IgM)

5 - Ag cell surface

1 - Antigen

Cytotoxic Ab

7 - Direct lysis especially via an activated complement enzyme cascade, as in the haemolysis encountered in blood transfusions

6 - The interaction of Ab (IgG or IgM) with a cell surface antigen causes cell destruction

Cytotoxic auto-antibodies are produced for unknown reasons against the glomerular basement membrane in **Goodpasture's syndrome**, against thyroid cells in **Hashimoto's disease** and against erythrocytes in **auto-immune haemolytic anaemia.** Sometimes, viruses and drugs may promote the production of cytotoxic antibodies.

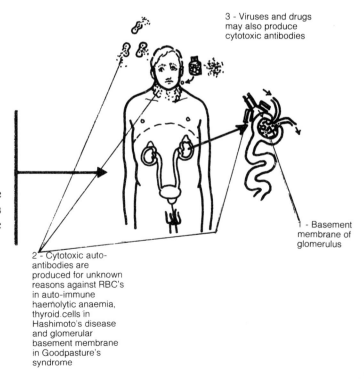

3 - Viruses and drugs may also produce cytotoxic antibodies

1 - Basement membrane of glomerulus

2 - Cytotoxic auto-antibodies are produced for unknown reasons against RBC's in auto-immune haemolytic anaemia, thyroid cells in Hashimoto's disease and glomerular basement membrane in Goodpasture's syndrome

1 - Ag-Ab complexes (equivalence) may mediate local or systemic damage

Ab

Ag Ag

Ab   **Ab**

Ag Ag

Ab

TYPE III - IMMUNE COMPLEX SENSITIVITY

Ag-Ab complexes may mediate local or systemic damage. When the **Ag-Ab** complexes form and there is an excess **Ab**, the **Ag** may be localised with an inflammatory response (Arthus reaction) and clinical syndromes may result – for example, in the lung where inhalation of dust from mouldy hay may cause an allergic alveolitis (farmer's lung).

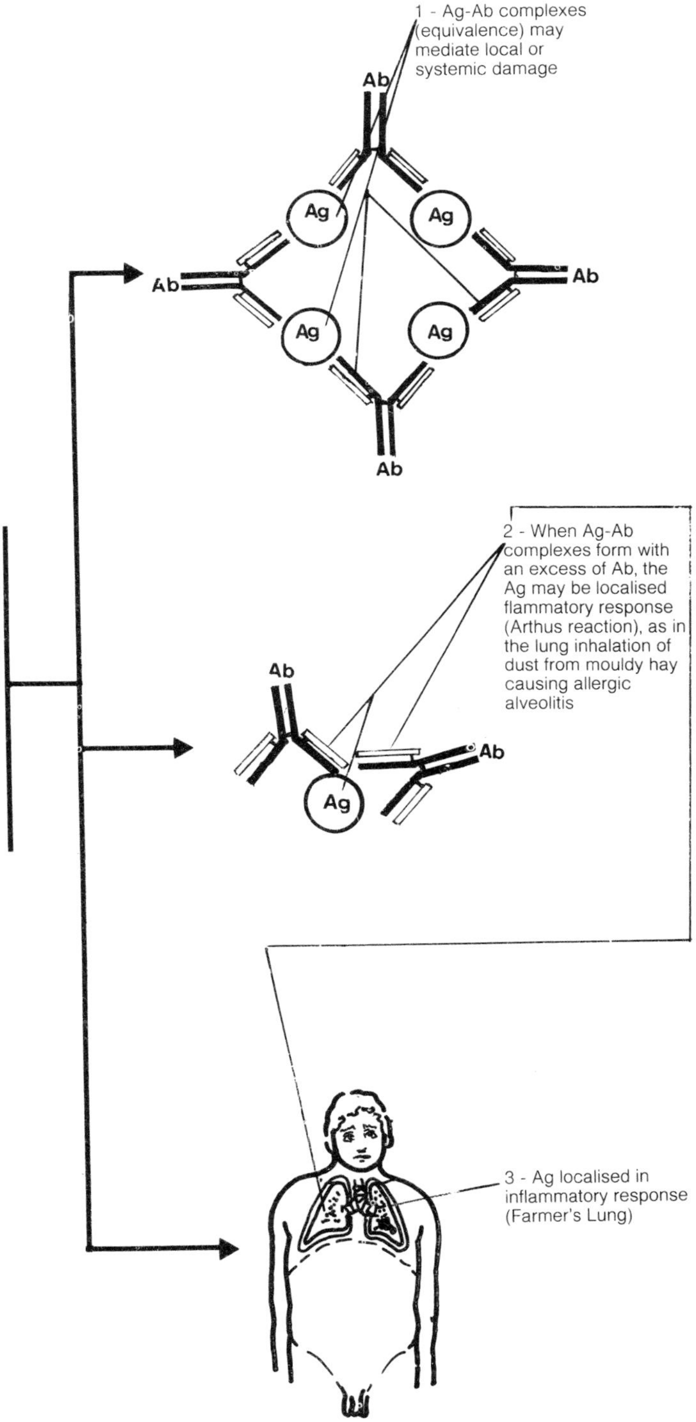

2 - When Ag-Ab complexes form with an excess of Ab, the Ag may be localised flammatory response (Arthus reaction), as in the lung inhalation of dust from mouldy hay causing allergic alveolitis

Ab

Ab

Ag

3 - Ag localised in inflammatory response (Farmer's Lung)

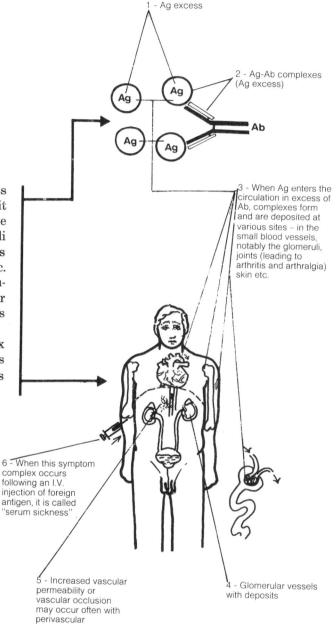

1 - Ag excess

2 - Ag-Ab complexes (Ag excess)

When **Ag** enters the circulation in excess of **Ab**, then the complexes form and deposit in various sites – predominantly in the small blood vessels, notably the glomeruli (leading to glomerulonephritis), joints (leading to arthralgia or arthritis), skin etc. Increased vascular permeability or vascular occlusion may occur and a perivascular inflammatory response (peri-arteritis) is common.

When this whole symptom complex occurs together following an intravenous administration of a foreign antigen, it is called "**serum sickeness**".

3 - When Ag enters the circulation in excess of Ab, complexes form and are deposited at various sites – in the small blood vessels, notably the glomeruli, joints (leading to arthritis and arthralgia) skin etc.

6 - When this symptom complex occurs following an I.V. injection of foreign antigen, it is called "serum sickness"

5 - Increased vascular permeability or vascular occlusion may occur often with perivascular inflammation

4 - Glomerular vessels with deposits

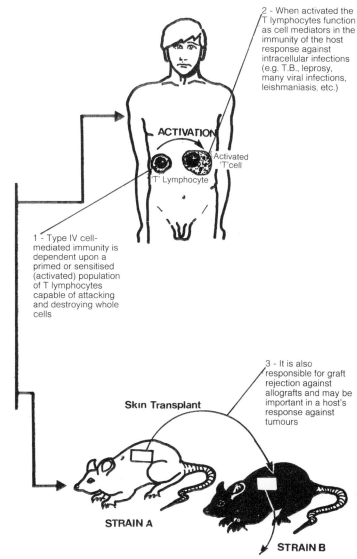

2 - When activated the T lymphocytes function as cell mediators in the immunity of the host response against intracellular infections (e.g. T.B., leprosy, many viral infections, leishmaniasis, etc.)

ACTIVATION

Activated 'T'cell

'T' Lymphocyte

1 - Type IV cell-mediated immunity is dependent upon a primed or sensitised (activated) population of T lymphocytes capable of attacking and destroying whole cells

3 - It is also responsible for graft rejection against allografts and may be important in a host's response against tumours

Skin Transplant

STRAIN A

STRAIN B

MOUSE TRANSPLANT REJECTION

TYPE IV - CELL MEDIATED SENSITIVITY

This type of sensitivity cannot be transferred between animals by humoral/serum antibodies. It is dependent upon a primed or sensitised population of **T** lymphocytes capable of attacking and destroying whole cells. Cell mediated immunity is a protective host response for destroying intracellular infections (e.g. T.B., leprosy, many viral infections, leishmaniasis etc.). It is also responsible for the most persistent graft rejection response raised against allografts and may be important in a host's response against tumours.

HYPERSENSITIVITY TYPE	ANTIGEN (EXAMPLES)	ANTIBODY CLASS	DISEASES/SYNDROME (EXAMPLES)
I (Anaphlylaxis)	Pollens Drug (e.g. aspirin) house dust mite	IgE	Anaphylaxis Urticaria Asthma Hay fever
II (Cytotoxic)	Auto-Ag (e.g. glomerular basement membrane) Virus Drug (e.g. sedormid)	IgG or IgM IgG or IgM IgG or IgM	Goodpasture's syndrome Hashimoto's disease Auto-immune haemolysis Post-measles encephalitis Ab-mediated thrombocytopenics
III (Immune Complex)	Auto-Ag (e.g. DNA) Virus Bacterium Protozoa Fungus Drug/Serum	IgG or IgM IgG or IgM IgG or IgM IgG or IgM IgG or IgM IgG or IgM	Systemic lupus erythematosus (S.L.E.) Viral hepatitis – systemic manifestations Post-streptococcal glomerulonephritis Malarial glomerulonephritis Fungal alveolitis Serum sickness Arthus reaction
IV (Cell Mediated)	Auto-Ag (e.g. Thyroglobulin, Thyroid microsomes) Virus Bacterium Protozoa Helminth	— — — — —	Hashimoto's disease Herpes Tuberculosis Leprosy Cutaneous leishmaniasis Schistosomiasis

Index